T0073199

COMMON SENSE IMPLEMENTATION OF QMS IN THE CLINICAL LABORATORY

A Software Guided Approach

COMMON SENSE IMPLEMENTATION OF QMS IN THE CLINICAL LABORATORY

M. Amano, R. Bredt, M. Colby, T. Freeman
Foreword by Hayato Miyachi, MD, PhD

World Scientific

NEW JERSEY • LONDON • SINGAPORE • BEIJING • SHANGHAI • HONG KONG • TAIPEI • CHENNAI • TOKYO

Published by

World Scientific Publishing Co. Pte. Ltd.
5 Toh Tuck Link, Singapore 596224
USA office: 27 Warren Street, Suite 401-402, Hackensack, NJ 07601
UK office: 57 Shelton Street, Covent Garden, London WC2H 9HE

Library of Congress Control Number: 2019951434

British Library Cataloguing-in-Publication Data
A catalogue record for this book is available from the British Library.

COMMON SENSE IMPLEMENTATION OF QMS IN THE CLINICAL LABORATORY
A Software Guided Approach

ISBN 978-981-121-247-5

For any available supplementary material, please visit
https://www.worldscientific.com/worldscibooks/10.1142/11612#t=suppl

Printed in Singapore

CONTENTS

FOREWORD

Quality Management Systems in the New Era of Clinical Laboratories

Hayato Miyachi, MD, PhD
Department of Laboratory Medicine, Tokai University School of Medicine

Clinical laboratories have been facing revolutionary changes. These changes include the clinical application of emerging technologies such as next-generation sequencing (NGS), new information technologies, and even integrated services based on the fourth industrial revolution, which includes areas like artificial intelligence, big data, and the Internet of Things.

Many laboratories struggle to understand these concepts and how they impact nearly everything they do. Implementing and maintaining Quality Management Systems (QMS) is certainly going to be central to driving understanding and, ultimately, creating change.

Every laboratory is different but the objectives of quality management are universal. These objectives are: creating and maintaining a safe environment, increasing productivity, and—most importantly—improving quality patient outcomes.

To reach these goals, laboratories must imbue QMS throughout their organization and involve each and every laboratory employee so that the lab culture understands that audits and accreditation are not the true or sole objective. Rather, the goal needs to be meaningful implementation of standards that have been painstakingly created by hundreds of top laboratory professionals from around the world. By the meaningful application of international standards, patients and physicians can and should have confidence in laboratory services.

Challenges abound. Laboratories face resource and human shortages. The reality, however, is that value can only be created through work. This work includes things like document creation and control but, perhaps most importantly, such work also must embrace education, quality meetings, user surveys, and real quality objectives. None of these things can occur in a vacuum because real

QMS requires transparency and accountability. Moreover, it requires leadership and commitment at all levels of the laboratory.

But, how can a laboratory be expected to build and maintain all the required standards? Fortunately, we have entered the information age where viable tools have become readily available. The first iteration of these new information tools consisted of document management systems, and they certainly helped organize documents and pass audits. But, one wonders, can a document management system alone really address the real spirit of compliance to QMS? Recently, however, a new kind of software tool has changed the paradigm for the better, as exemplified by LEAP Software. LEAP's objectives are to help laboratory leaders effectively build and run systems in accordance with international standards, to involve the entire laboratory in the process, and to ensure that the actionable maintenance of QMS standards occurs, on time, and in a meaningful fashion. LEAP can help managers understand all aspects of their QMS at a single glance and react to information such as non-conformities in real time.

It is my hope that LEAP, and this book, represent a real first step towards smart QMS based on the fourth industrial revolution and the new era of clinical laboratory medicine. Both products demonstrate clearly and comprehensively how new technologies can enable laboratory management to improve quality and support the best levels of patient care, which is, of course, our shared and ultimate goal.

BACKGROUND AND INTRODUCTION

About LEAP

LEAP is a cloud-based software system designed to help clinical laboratories meaningfully gain and maintain compliance to established Quality Management Systems (QMS). As of this writing, LEAP has been optimized for ISO 15189 and The College of American Pathologists (CAP) accreditation programs. LEAP provides for parallel compliance management for both ISO and CAP programs in a single platform. LEAP's primary objective is to extract intrinsic value from the process and results of QMS by involving the entire laboratory staff and guiding them through the building and maintenance of standards in a highly transparent and accountable way.

This book is designed to be used in conjunction with LEAP or equivalent software systems.

Introduction

"It is all just common sense." This short phrase has been this author's (Mark Colby) mantra for over 30 years of helping clinical laboratories gain and maintain QMS. Going one step further, my first rule in implementing QMS is always: "If you don't understand why you're doing something—don't do it!"

Both of these pieces of advice typically earn me strange looks from clients, especially highly trained quality managers who feel hurt that all their time spent acquiring highly technical skills and understanding the supporting quality theories and advanced analytical methods are being challenged. This is not my intent; quite the contrary. Having a skilled quality manager is, in my opinion, a cornerstone to driving quality processes. The issue, however, is that the majority of laboratory employees are not highly skilled quality managers. Moreover, these non-specialized quality people are, in fact, the ones who ultimately determine the level of quality. Thus, their participation is critical to achieve the true intent of *quality*, which is, of course, to increase productivity, safety and most importantly: the quality of patient outcomes.

Maintaining compliance to various standards is a reality for most people working in a clinical lab. There is, however, a big difference between maintaining the rule vs. the spirit of any QMS. Maintaining rules because they are, well, rules, results in too much paper and a lot of work. Maintaining the spirit of compliance results in intrinsic value.

In my experience, for core laboratory employees to maintain the spirit of compliance, the key factor is for people to truly understand why they're doing things. And, in the end, for them to understand *why* they're doing things, they need to understand the 'common sense' nature that can be found at the core of almost all QMS processes.

Once laboratory staff understand the true, common-sense intent of a QMS standard, the likelihood of incorporating these standards into their day-to-day work increases dramatically. With time, these standards become second-nature and a habit. This is when the magic happens. And this is when laboratories and their users get the benefits of all the work and investment.

But, you may ask, how can anyone call nearly all QMS processes common sense? The answer is simple: you need to ask yourself two questions. First, what are the potential risks if I don't do a particular QMS task? Second, what are the benefits of doing that QMS task? I believe you'll find that, when critically examining nearly all QMS standards, there are affirmative answers to each of these questions. If you understand this, it qualifies for my common-sense designation.

As mentioned above, it is also my opinion that if you don't understand the common-sense rationale for implementing and maintaining any particular standard, you shouldn't do it. Of course, this comes with the caveat that ignoring standards can lead to lapses in regulatory compliance, which can then in turn lead to all sorts of trouble. Regardless, I stand by my view that implementing a standard that is ill-understood is a waste of time and money and basically a meaningless exercise. Thus, the objective needs to be one of seeking understanding through discussion and, if necessary, seeking outside advice. If understanding remains elusive, my next recommendation is to ask your auditors and inspectors for advice. If they can't address the question of why this is important, the final step is to challenge the particular standard at the source. Both CAP and most ISO-notified bodies have established processes for challenging standards and it is an important part of their QMS processes—so never be shy about asking them why a particular standard is necessary.

A QMS is much more than merely the rote performance of monitors and tasks. An organization that only repeats these tasks will find quality management to be cumbersome, burdensome, resource-intensive, time consuming, and not very useful.

Instead, the best quality systems adopt a dynamic approach to building, assuring, and maintaining quality. Organizations that critically monitor their quality systems, adapt to external changes and nonconformities, discontinue unneeded monitors, and solicit staff and customer input for their QMS are ultimately more successful at improving quality.

Some regulatory requirements may seem similar to aspects of a QMS. They are put into place by an individual laboratory to satisfy the standards for external entities. While these often must be done to satisfy governmental or other regulatory bodies, they should not entirely substitute for an individual laboratory QMS. Where quality is concerned, one size does not fit all.

For each standard in each LEAP FOS overview there is a section dedicated to "why is this important." While each laboratory is different, this is a generic explanation as to what might happen if you don't undertake the standard(s) and what positive things might come out of undertaking it/them. In other words: why it's just common sense.

The QMS Issues

There are several things that essentially guarantee that your laboratory will spend a great deal of time and money on QMS and receive very little except a pretty certificate for all the efforts. These are:

1) Isolated Quality Manager(s): I am always saddened when I examine a laboratory and find the quality manager stuck alone in a corner while the people doing the 'real work' ignore them. To achieve intrinsic value, *everyone* needs to be involved in quality processes. In the paper-based world of the past, this was usually just a fantasy. In today's digital world and with the right tools and leadership, this objective can actually become a reality. The quality manager must be the conductor, however, while everyone else needs to be responsible for making the music.

2) Powerless Quality Manager(s): Quality managers can only be effective if they have direct-line authority to the laboratory director or those who can institute change. An organization with isolated quality managers who report to the departments, rather than centrally, runs the risk of having an ineffective quality system. Nonconformities may not be examined, may be overlooked, and may not be acted upon if the reporting is only within the monitored department.

3) Actionable vs. Non-actionable: Actionable items are things requiring a defined action performed at certain intervals. Few of these actions are particularly difficult, but the totality of them makes the QMS gears turn and accrues value. Non-actionable items are things that are more conceptual in nature and may be incorporated in your policies, but require no specific action and leave no tangible evidence. Placing a non-quality-trained person in charge of a non-actionable item will lead to frustration and confusion (or the ignoring of important issues) instead of a focus on processes requiring specific actions and leaving evidence of these actions.

4) Transparency and Accountability: The bane of any QMS are the piles of documents, assignments, and processes that end up buried, unused, and unchecked. Again, in the paper-based world of the past, creating accountable and transparent systems was a monumental task requiring tremendous amounts of management effort. In today's digital world, however, with the right tools and effective management oversight, not only can transparent and accountable processes be implemented and maintained effectively, from a management perspective this can also be done nearly effortlessly.

In stark contrast to greater ease for management, these improvements in accountability and transparency require that those assigned to actionable projects must be highly vigilant. At first, this will seem like even more work. In time, however, these processes will become second nature. Then, and only then, the laboratory can finally begin to experience the intended realized intrinsic value.

5) Monitors without Thresholds: There is not much point to monitoring an activity or performance if there is no established threshold for action. Goals and targets must be set which, if not met, will trigger some action by the quality system. The best thresholds are ones based on external requirements such as customer needs or industry standards. If these don't exist, the laboratory may establish thresholds based on its own standards and develop and revise these over time. Ask yourselves this question: "If we don't have a target for this monitor, then why are we monitoring it?"

6) Useless Monitors: Nothing detracts more from an organization's quality efforts than the rote repetition of monitors without critical analysis. If a monitor has a threshold of 95% and the laboratory is always well above that goal, is the lab truly getting the most out of all the time and resources spent on performing that monitor? Individual monitors, like the overall QMS, should be critically reviewed and adjusted if necessary. Perhaps the laboratory should increase the threshold to 98%. If it is not a regulatory requirement, perhaps the laboratory should cease this monitor and choose a new one that's more beneficial to improving quality.

7) The Useless Quality Manual: Nothing is sadder than a well-written and beautifully formatted—and lonely—quality manual. The tendency for quality manuals to be used only during inspections or audits is so prevalent, I believe their use should be abandoned. Rather, through modern, available, digital systems, the quality manual should not be confined to a single document but instead be something that permeates all aspects of laboratory testing.

8) Inspection Cycle Blues: "Oh my! The inspection is next month!" No one sleeps, documents are memorialized. Then the inspection occurs and deficiencies are corrected. And then the process gets repeated. In the interim until the next inspection, nothing much happens until this frenzied process starts yet again. Quality is and should be a continuous process. An inspection is not the time to perform the process but instead is merely the time for an assessment of that process.

It is a commonly known and seldom-discussed fact that this cycle occurs in most laboratories to varying degrees. Once again, however, this is the 21st century and things don't have to be this way anymore. The inspection-cycle blues is completely fixable through the implementation and use of modern digital tools that monitor and document ongoing compliance. The once-dirty secret has now been exposed.

LEAP Software

For a complete tutorial and specifications see: http://cgikk.com/en/leap.html

To understand LEAP software, and therefore understand this document, you need to comprehend the concept behind the Family of Standards, or what we refer to as 'FOS.'

Family of Standards (FOS): The core component of LEAP is the logical grouping of manageable-sized standards into something we call an FOS. Each FOS is designed to create a bite-sized group of rules (standards) requiring creation and maintenance. These groupings, while derived from the standards and guidelines, are the invention/creation of a QMS consulting company called CGI.

The FOS Process Structure

All FOS are structured identically. Therefore, the process of implementing the FOS QMS components and the ongoing maintenance after implementation are identical. Once a laboratory staff member knows how to implement one FOS, they will know how to implement them all. The process structure for each FOS is as follows: (Please note that we have used a simplified sample of temperature monitoring as an example to make the concept easier to understand.).

The CAP or ISO Standard / Guidelines

"Periodically Monitor Temperature."

Gap Analysis Questions

"Do you periodically monitor and record temperature?"

Policy for Customization

"The laboratory will periodically monitor and record temperature."

SOP for Customization

"The laboratory will monitor temperature daily and input the recordings on the temperature log."

FOS Maintenance Confirmation

"Upload all Temperature Logs into LEAP every month."

Components of Each FOS Content Library: Each FOS contains the following tools:

a) An overview document consisting of the original standards and guidelines followed by a commentary. This commentary breaks down and explains the common-sense nature of the FOS, the risks associated with non-compliance, and the benefits of compliance.

b) An education module that explains the intent and how to comply with all components of the FOS.

c) Templates of all policies and procedures and associated document requirements.

d) Samples of all templates showing what they need to look like once they are placed into service.

5 Steps of Building Compliance for Each FOS

In a case where you designate any component of an FOS not to be in compliance, LEAP will create a project for you whereby you assign managers and due dates. This requires that the laboratory undertakes and completes five tasks. These tasks are designed to make both the project leaders and everyone throughout the organization *think*. These five tasks are:

Task 1) Download and customize templates and request management approval.

Task 2) Ensure all stakeholders review the materials approved in Task 1.

Task 3) Create a budget, as necessary.

Task 4) Assign FOS maintenance managers and QMS maintenance intervals, and…

Task 5) Compile all completed materials into the inspection-ready, Master Evidence Folder (MEF).

In the case your gap analysis determines your laboratory is already in compliance with the FOS, the project will only consist of two tasks:

Task 4) Assign FOS maintenance managers and QMS maintenance intervals, and...

Task 5) Compile all completed materials into the inspection-ready, Master Evidence Folder (MEF).

Maintaining the Completed FOS

Once an FOS is completed, it immediately goes into maintenance mode. FOS maintenance managers will receive e-mails and can manage all QMS activities on their personalized MY MAINTENANCE TASKS page. The quality manger and laboratory management will be notified immediately for corrective action if any aspect of your QMS goes out of compliance.

Using FOS to Create a Cohesive QMS Process

The principle behind LEAP is to complete each FOS one at a time using a process that inculcates individual and organizational understanding and cements maintenance protocols for all actionable items. Think of each FOS as a brick or a building block. As each brick is laid, it's as if the laboratory's QMS rises one brick at a time until the entire QMS structure is complete—with each FOS active and functioning.

Of course, however, bricks stacked loosely and not bonded to each other lack strength. For your QMS brick house, time is the mortar that ties all the bricks together. As all FOS (bricks) are maintained and ultimately become a shared habit, the mortar between the bricks thickens and cures and becomes the foundation of your organization.

MY TASKS

Ultimately, value is only achieved by doing work, which means individuals must perform and complete an organized and coordinated set of specific tasks at designated intervals. A successful QMS requires that hundreds or even thousands of these tasks must be completed by dozens or even hundreds of people. While the laboratory director or quality manager needs to understand the big picture, the laboratory rank and file need to focus on their individual responsibilities. This is why LEAP provides a MY TASKS view customized to each individual for the development of QMS processes, and a MY MAINTENANCE TASKS view customized for each individual or the maintenance of all QMS processes.

Automated Self Audits

You can set your LEAP system to audit your entire organization yearly, or you can set LEAP to audit each department, spreading the audit process over time. Regardless of method, we suggest that you audit your systems at least once a year.

The automated self-audit process is simple. Upon initiating an audit, all of the green Master Evidence Folders (MEF) as well as their associated project folders turn gray. The project managers are then notified and have 30 days to complete the audit, initiate changes, and receive approval from a superior. Regular self audits confirm and strengthen each FOS as well as the mortar that binds them.

CAP vs. ISO

The concepts in managing QMS for both CAP and ISO within LEAP are identical. The reason we have chosen to highlight the ISO standard in this document is because it is more brief than CAP, lacking specific technical requirements for each technical specialty. Furthermore, by being more general, ISO tends to require expert opinion for application. The CAP standards, on the other hand, are very specific and well defined within CAP's checklist.

In the case of CAP, under CAP license, LEAP has used the exact text from the CAP checklist and guidance documentation. ISO, however, requires interpretation, or what might more aptly be called an 'opinion.' Therefore, for ISO, the suggested policies and procedures reflect the opinion of this author(s).

Suggested Schedule

While the schedule for implementing your QMS processes may vary, the following is a guide to give you some reference on navigating the process in a logical, step-by-step order. Note that, as soon as projects are completed, the QMS maintenance phase begins.

Numbers indicate months to completion

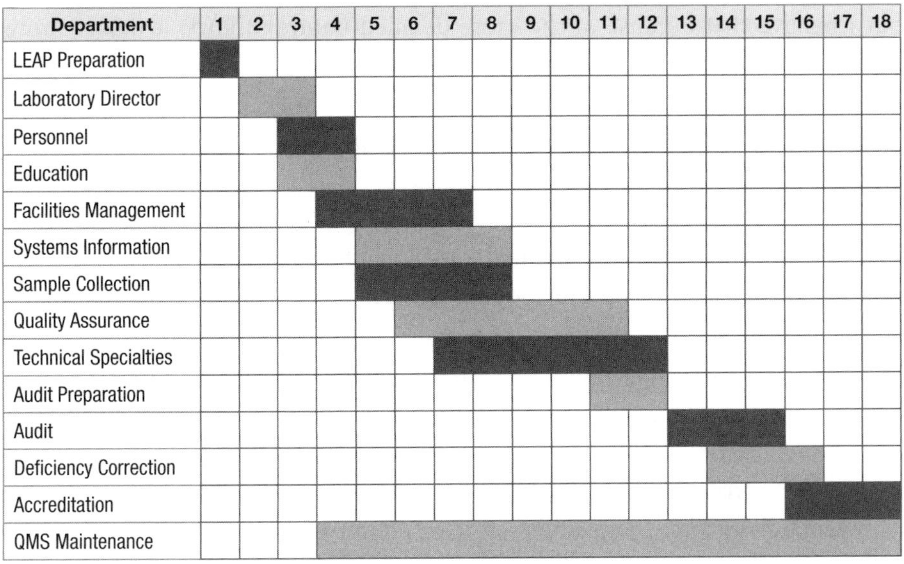

Department	1	2	3	4	5	6	7	8	9	10	11	12	13	14	15	16	17	18
LEAP Preparation																		
Laboratory Director																		
Personnel																		
Education																		
Facilities Management																		
Systems Information																		
Sample Collection																		
Quality Assurance																		
Technical Specialties																		
Audit Preparation																		
Audit																		
Deficiency Correction																		
Accreditation																		
QMS Maintenance																		

Implementing Both CAP and ISO

Some laboratories may choose to implement both CAP and ISO standards. In many cases, laboratories deal with this duality by maintaining two separate quality systems and thus, in my opinion, creating a confusing mosaic of processes which defeat the objective of creating a common-sense actionable quality environment.

LEAP allows your laboratory to implement both CAP and ISO into one quality environment. This is done by activating two departments for each technical area. For example, imagine you have both a CAP clinical chemistry department and ISO clinical chemistry department. As such, you will need to designate either CAP or ISO as the primary standard and complete all FOSs within that department. Next, you will complete the 'secondary' department, referencing materials in the primary department rather than duplicating them. Issues that are not satisfied in the primary department are created and maintained in the secondary department. This allows the lab staff and auditors/inspectors to seamlessly build, monitor, and maintain dual quality environments in a single system without duplication.

There may be some debate about whether CAP or ISO should take precedence, but I believe that because of the more detailed nature of CAP, it makes more sense to designate CAP as the primary standard.

Technical Departments Included in the CAP version of LEAP

The following technical departments are included in the LEAP software. As new technical specialties are introduced by CAP additional departments will be added.

Anatomic Pathology
Chemistry and Toxicology
Flow Cytometry
Forensic Drug Testing
Hematology and Coagulation
Immunology
Microbiology
Molecular Pathology
Clinical Biochemical Genetics
Cytogenetics
Cytopathology
Histocompatibility
Point-of-Care Testing
Reproductive Laboratory
Transfusion Medicine
Urinalysis

Leadership

I have good news and bad news. The good news is that LEAP, once initiated, will manage all of your QMS processes seamlessly and create near total accountability and transparency with little effort or time. The bad news is that, without leadership and oversight by laboratory management, the only thing using LEAP will accomplish is to provide ample evidence that the laboratory operates out of compliance.

To successfully operate your QMS using LEAP, people must be assigned to monitor the QMS dashboards and *act* when problems are sighted. The color yellow indicates caution and we recommend that you contact the relevant person if they are nearing a deadline. Your leaders need to instill a culture in which red-colored designations are considered unacceptable performance.

Your LEAP QMS leaders also need to watch for changes in your organization and reappoint the maintenance task managers and team members when staff are transferred, become ill, or leave for other reasons.

Managing Inspections

After you have completed building your QMS and have used LEAP to maintain these systems, I encourage you to offer auditors and inspectors access to your LEAP account by giving them temporary Auditors Access permissions about a month prior to the inspection. This will give the auditor or inspector full access to view LEAP's documents and dig into the processes used to develop these processes. They will have read-only permissions, but can leave comments in the evidence folders. This will make for a more productive inspection process. Prior document access allows a more efficient use of on-site assessment time and may allow for an initial gap analysis prior to the on-site assessment.

The Organization of this Document

This document is organized by department. Each department will have multiple FOS (see above). Each FOS will have the following components: a) FOS Overview; b) Recommended Policies; c) Procedure Template; d) List of other materials located within LEAP.

LEAP users will be guided through the following steps in chronologic order. This is the same order as outlined:

1) QMS Process Preparation
2) Laboratory Director
3) Personnel
4) Facilities
5) Information Management
6) Sample Collection
7) Quality Assurance
8) Technical Specialties
9) Audit Preparation

The Quality Manual

It is this author's opinion that the LEAP system and supporting polices and documentation meet all of the regulatory requirements of a quality manual and can actually replace a quality manual. However, we do recognize there are different opinions on this matter, so there is an opportunity to create a quality manual as the final FOS, as found within the Quality Assurance Department. This template should be populated with content components built prior to completing the quality manual.

If you do choose to maintain a quality manual, you will need to manually update this document as changes get made within LEAP. Again, treating LEAP as your quality manual is likely the best decision. Defending this position with an auditor or inspector will consist on explaining that a quality manual is a static document while LEAP represents an ongoing and more organic process driving real and value-added QMS processes.

Representative Sample of a Policy and Procedure

The LEAP process provides an overview of each FOS designed to give your laboratory insight about how and why the standards need to be implemented. It also has a sample policy and procedure and any log sheets or other materials you will be required to build and maintain. It is important to note that these materials are generic and typically require significant customization to meet the unique needs of your laboratory. You are encouraged to review the overview, educational materials, sample policy and procedure, and other logs or manuals, thereafter, think about how these can be modified to best meet your needs. LEAP has indicated specific areas that will require customization. This includes inserting names of responsible persons, intervals of certain activities and referencing associated documentation such as log sheets and manuals that are typically also included in LEAP.

In the heat of building your QMS, there may be the temptation to use the policies, procedures, and other supporting materials without considering your needs. An even more problematic practice will be to use the materials without even reading them. Needless to say, this will lead to a 'garbage-in-garbage out' situation and will lead to ineffective QMS processes.

Sample: Quality Indicators Policy and Procedure

POLICIES

1) The laboratory must establish quality indicators to monitor and evaluate performance throughout critical aspects of pre-examination, examination and post-examination processes.

2) The laboratory must plan the process of monitoring quality indicators, which includes establishing objectives, methodology, interpretation, limits, action plan, and duration of measurement.

3) The laboratory must periodically review the indicators to ensure their continued appropriateness.

4) The laboratory, in consultation with the users, must establish turnaround times for each of its examinations that reflect clinical needs.

5) The laboratory must periodically evaluate whether or not it is meeting the established turnaround times.

PROCEDURES

Identifying and Establishing Quality Indicators

1) The laboratory must develop and maintain "Laboratory-wide" Quality Indicators to monitor issues affecting the entire laboratory as well as "Department specific" Quality Indicators that affect only the individual department.

2) The following materials can be used to identify relevant Quality Indicators.
   a. Customer Complaint Logs
   b. Nonconformity Event Investigation Logs
   c. Inquiry Logs
   d. Quality Control Data
   e. Customer Survey Data
   f. Employee Survey Data
   g. Quality Meeting Minutes
   h. Local or regional requirements
   i. Requirements of ISO standards or accrediting organization requirements
   j. Other materials and information available to the laboratory

3) While discussion on the above topics should be held during the quality meeting with minutes noted in the **"Quality Meeting Minutes" (ID: QA013-XXX-XXX)**, the quality manager will be responsible for managing the Quality Indicators identified during the meeting in a form of a **"Quality Indicator Worksheet" (ID: DIR06-XXX-XXX)**. The form should include specific objectives and the association to the laboratory's quality objectives. There should be **at least three (3)** active "Laboratory-wide" and "Department specific" Quality Indicators respectively.

4) Each Quality Indicator must have quantifiable indices that must be defined, monitored, and recorded.

5) LEAP Maintenance Protocol for this step will be set for **quarterly** review to ensure that the quality indicators are properly monitored using the quantifiable indices and any other relevant information. This review should include graph representation of the indices where applicable.

Establishing Performance Thresholds for Each Quality Indicator

1) Each Quality Indicator should also be associated with a goal or threshold for action. Indicators for which the threshold is not met should trigger action by the laboratory. Repeated missing of performance targets **must** trigger action by the laboratory. These actions should be noted in the **"Quality Indicator Worksheet" (ID: DIR06-XXX-XXX)**. Threshold or targets may be based upon user needs, regulations, accrediting organization requirements, employee recommendations, or prior laboratory experience. Possible action in response to unmet threshold is:
   a. Initiating a quality project
   b. Reviewing and modifying the performance goal
   c. Continuing the monitor for another cycle (this must be documented, should not be over-utilized, and should not be repeatedly used for the same indicator).

2) LEAP Maintenance Protocol for this step will be set for **quarterly** review to ensure that the performance threshold is appropriate and being met.

Periodic Review of Quality Indicators

1) The continued applicability of each indicator should be reviewed **annually**. Indicators that are continuously met should be discontinued (unless required by external requirements) and replaced with other indicators that can have a greater impact on quality.

Materials accessible within LEAP

- Quality Indicators Worksheet (Template)
- Quality Indicators Worksheet (Sample)
- Quality Indicators Examples

QUALITY INDICATOR (Template)

<table>
<tr><td colspan="2">Objectives</td></tr>
<tr><td colspan="2">Definition</td></tr>
<tr><td>Data Collection Methods</td><td rowspan="2">Data Presentation: Quality Indicator Graph</td></tr>
<tr><td>Action Threshold / Target</td></tr>
<tr><td colspan="2">Interpretation</td></tr>
<tr><td colspan="2">Limitations to Interpretation</td></tr>
<tr><td colspan="2">Action Plans for Various Outcomes and Interpretations</td></tr>
<tr><td>Signature</td><td></td></tr>
</table>

QUALITY INDICATOR (Sample 1)

NGS Tests Ordered (June)

Objectives

Increase physician awareness of the availability and utility of NGS testing to increase the effectiveness of cancer diagnosis and patient outcomes.

Background

The number of NGS testings ordered is well below average when compared to inter-system data and national averages. This appears to be due to the lack of physician awareness.

Data Collection Methods

The number of NGS tests ordered will be counted on a monthly basis and placed in a graph.

Action Threshold / Target

Increase in the number of NGS tests ordered to reflect the system average of 30 per month from the current 2 per month.

Data Presentation: Quality Indicator Graph

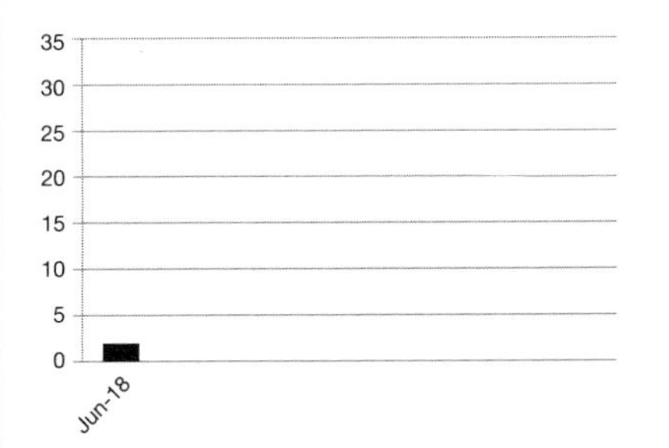

Interpretation

Number of tests reported

Limitations to Interpretation

None

Summary

Jun. 01, 2018 The manufacturer will be asked to perform a physician in-service education program. This will be followed by offering an e-learning program offered on the laboratory's website. We will also interact with the pharmacy and request they inform physicians about the availability and utility of NGS testing when associated with drugs that are being prescribed. We will recommend to administration that NGS testing be included on diagnosis and treatment protocols.

Signature	*Laboratory Director* *Mark Colby* *Jun. 15, 2018*

QUALITY INDICATOR (Sample 2)

NGS Tests Ordered (September)

Objectives

Increase physician awareness of the availability and utility of NGS testing to increase the effectiveness of cancer diagnosis and patient outcomes.

Background

The number of NGS testings ordered is well below average when compared to inter-system data and national averages. This appears to be due to the lack of physician awareness.

Data Collection Methods

The number of NGS tests ordered will be counted on a monthly basis and placed in a graph.

Action Threshold / Target

Increase in the number of NGS tests ordered to reflect the system average of 30 per month from the current 2 per month.

Data Presentation: Quality Indicator Graph

NGS Tests Ordered

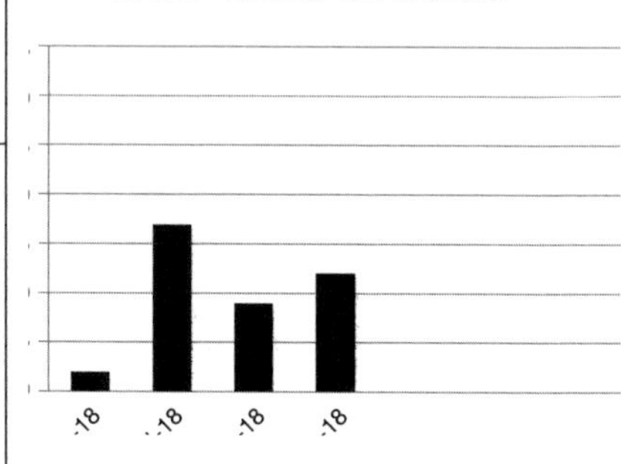

Interpretation

Number of tests reported

Limitations to Interpretation

None

Summary

Sep. 01, 2018 While orders for NGS testing have increased compared to June, this has not been consistent. We will send out notifications to physicians who participated in the manufacturer's in-service education program as well as the e-learning program to remind them of the benefits of NGS testing.

Signature	*Laboratory Director* *Mark Colby* *Sep. 15, 2018*

QUALITY INDICATOR (Sample 3)

NGS Tests Ordered (December)

Objectives

Increase physician awareness of the availability and utility of NGS testing to increase the effectiveness of cancer diagnosis and patient outcomes.

Background

The number of NGS testing ordered is well below average when compared to inter-system data and national averages. This appears to be due to the lack of physician awareness.

Data Collection Methods

The number of NGS tests ordered will be counted on a monthly basis and placed in a graph.

Action Threshold / Target

Increase in the number of NGS tests ordered to reflect the system average of 30 per month from the current 2 per month.

Data Presentation: Quality Indicator Graph

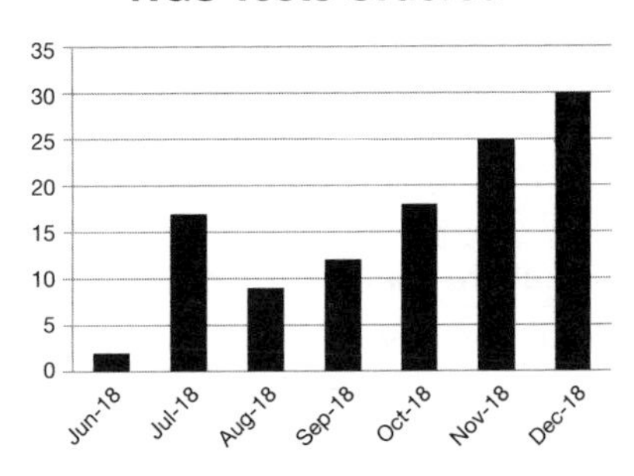

Interpretation

Number of tests reported

Limitations to Interpretation

None

Summary

Dec. 01, 2018 Objectives have been met, but we will continue monitoring the numbers to ensure that a constant order of NGS testing.

Signature

Laboratory Director
Mark Colby
Dec. 01, 2018

QUALITY INDICATOR (Examples)

System-related Quality Indicators
Cost/benefit ratio (e.g. cost of laboratory test per patient outcome)
Customer satisfaction—patient or physician satisfaction with laboratory services
Diabetes monitoring (e.g. percentage of diabetics with annual hemoglobin A1c results)
Safety (e.g. needlestick injury occurrences)
Staff competency (e.g. monitoring technologists' ability to detect a known sample)
Verification of physicians' orders to point-of-care examinations

Public Health-related Quality Indicators
Number of nursing home residents with antibiotic-resistant infections

Pre-Examination-related Quality Indicators
Accuracy of patient identification
Adequacy and accuracy of sample information
Appropriateness of bone marrow samples
Appropriateness of sample container
Blood culture contamination rate
Chain-of-custody
Correct sample labeling (incl. mislabeled and unlabeled specimens)
Accuracy and appropriateness of requisition forms
Examination utilization by physicians for best care
Identification of inpatients not wearing wristbands
Number of unsatisfactory cervicovaginal cytology samples (e.g. obscuring factors, poor cellularity)
Ordered examination is appropriate for patient care
Patient consent appropriately collected
Patients' satisfaction with phlebotomy services
Phlebotomy success
Physician's written order with every sample
Preparation of patient for sample collection
Requisition monitoring for correct examination ordering
Requisition monitoring for correct ordering physician entry
Sample delivery times
Sample integrity
Sample quantity

Sample transportation
Timing of sample collection
Urine culture contamination rate

Examination-related Quality Indicators
Accuracy and timeliness of bone marrow reports
Accuracy of point-of-care testing
Cervical cytology/biopsy correlation
Comparison of "abnormal" rates and error rates for cervicovaginal samples by cytologist
Competency of personnel
Concordance for surgical pathology cases reviewed elsewhere
Correlation of fine-needle biopsy diagnosis with "final" diagnosis, by selected organ system
Effectiveness of "rules" to detect abnormal samples
External quality assurance (EQA)
Frozen section discordance
Investigation of examination failures in cytogenetics
Investigation of instrument "flagged" results
Laboratory injuries or accidents
QC process
Sample contamination
Surgical pathology slide review program
Time to result availability
Vacancy of technical staff

Post-Examination-related Quality Indicators
Adequacy of information for interpretation of laboratory examinations
Autoverification errors
Client satisfaction audits
Consistency of critical values reporting
Critical value reporting
Major corrections to surgical specifically with phlebotomy services
Proportion of corrected reports
Report delivery turnaround time
Result reporting accuracy
Review and approvals are evident

Turnaround Time-related Quality Indicators
Autopsy final report turnaround time
Compliance with internal turnaround time standards for emergency department stat examinations
Compliance with turnaround time standards promulgated by accrediting agencies and clinical professional societies
Cytology turnaround time
Frozen section turnaround time
Special chemistry turnaround time for cardiac injury markers and alcohol levels

Summary

LEAP represents a fundamentally new way of approaching laboratory QMS. LEAP allows you to build and maintain QMS from the bottom up, and at the same time provide transparency and accountability from the top down. It is a fully integrated system with project management, content, and education, all broken up into bite-sized, manageable pieces that allows your entire team to be a functional part of QMS. LEAP will allow each user to process and think about the information individually and within the organization as a whole, eventually transforming your QMS into a shared habit. The objective is to achieve intrinsic value in the form of increased productivity, safety, and to optimize the laboratory's role in advancing quality patient outcomes.

Okay. It is now time to get into the nitty-gritty as we examine each ISO 15189 standard. I hope you find it useful and helps you build a safe, productive clinical laboratory and contributes to the best patient outcomes possible!

Sincerely Yours,

Mark Colby
Co-Author
Common Sense Implementation of QMS in a Clinical Laboratory: a software guided approach

INITIAL PREPARATION

FOS: Initial QMS Process Preparation

To begin implementing your laboratory QMS system using LEAP, you will need to contract with CGI or a licensed LEAP reseller. LEAP may also be available under different brand names.

Upon obtaining your LEAP license, you will be asked to provide certain information including the names and email addresses of everyone in your laboratory who will use LEAP, what technical departments you will want activated, and if you want to use LEAP to implement ISO, CAP, or both. You will be provided with a survey in the form of an Excel file by the seller.

The next step will be for your laboratory to adopt certain policies. These policies are listed in this department.

Why being in compliance with this FOS is important:

LEAP is a tool and, like any tool, it is only as effective as the people using it. Failing to implement the policies and procedures to set up LEAP will lead to frustration from the users and ineffective implementation and maintenance of your QMS. Like any tool, the use of LEAP will require practice. The better your team gets at using LEAP, the move effective your QMS implementation will be.

Materials Included In This FOS
• Initial QMS Process Preparation Policies and Procedures

FOS: Education Set Up

Education is an important and ongoing requirement for QMS in general. In LEAP, there are two kinds of education. The first involves Education Modules found within the **FOS Content Library**. The second includes document review of all materials created in Task 1, particularly the policies and procedures.

In Task 2, LEAP allows you to select documents from Task 1 that need to be reviewed by certain members in the laboratory. Once Task 2 is set up, LEAP will send an email notification to all relevant personnel with a link that will take the person(s) directly to the folder containing the documents that require review. Once the person(s) finish reviewing the document, they will click "Review Complete" and the system will keep a record of this. Project Managers and above also have the ability to send additional reminders to person(s) who have not completed their reviews on time.

The laboratory can decide to have all education managed centrally by either one person or groups of people (e.g., by setting up an education department or by the quality assurance department or this education can be managed by each department manager. There are advantages to both methods, and the choice of methods will depend primarily upon the size and complexity of your laboratory, i.e., a very large laboratory will likely need to manage education on a department basis.

There is also a hybrid option, whereby LEAP Education Modules are managed centrally but the review of Task 1 materials is managed at the department level. Regardless of the option selected, the laboratory should determine which department and person supervises the education and documentation.

Why being in compliance with this FOS is important:

Laboratory staff can only be reasonably expected to conform to QMS processes if they understand them. Lack of implementing an effective education process will create misunderstandings and frustration at all levels. This can lead to errors in the process and accidents as well as introduce unwanted variability into test results and decreases the level of patient care. Successfully implementing an education program will ensure that people understand their role in the QMS process, the importance of QMS overall, their role in improving and assuring quality, ensuring that they adhere to both the letter and spirit of QMS. This will bring value in the form of increased productivity, safety, and quality patient outcomes.

Materials Included In This FOS
• LEAP Education Set up Policies and Procedures
• Education Delegation Worksheet

LABORATORY DIRECTOR

FOS: Document Control / ISO 4.3

Please note that all text noted in shaded boxes are actual ISO **requirements**.

4.3 Document Control

The laboratory shall control documents required by the quality management system and shall ensure that unintended use of any obsolete documents is prevented.

NOTE 1: Documents that should be considered for document control are those that may vary based on change in versions or time. Examples include policy statements, instructions for use, flow charts, procedures, specifications, forms, calibration tables, biological reference intervals and their origins, charts, posters, notices, memoranda, software documentation, drawings, plans, agreements, and documents of external origin such as regulations, standards and textbooks from which examination procedures are taken.

NOTE 2: Records contain information from a particular point in time stating results achieved or providing evidence of activities performed and are maintained according to the requirements given in 4.13, Control of Records.

The laboratory shall have a documented procedure to ensure that the following conditions are met:

a) All documents, including those maintained in a computerized system, issued as part of the quality management system are reviewed and approved by authorized personnel before issue.
b) All documents are identified to include:
   - A title
   - A unique identifier on each page
   - The date of the current edition and/or edition number
   - Page number to total number of pages (e.g., "Page 1 of 5", "Page 2 of 5")
   - Authority for issue

NOTE: "Edition" is used to mean one of a number of printings issued at separate times that incorporates alterations and amendments. "Edition" can be regarded as synonymous with "revision" or "version".

c) Current authorized editions and their distributions are identified by means of a list (e.g., document register, log or master index).
d) Only current, authorized editions of applicable documents are available at point of use.
e) Where a laboratory's document control system allows for the amendment of documents by hand, pending the re-issue of documents, the procedures and authorities for such amendments are defined, amendments are clearly marked, initialized and dated, and a revised document is issued within a specified time period.
f) Changes to documents are identified.
g) Documents remain legible.
h) Documents are periodically reviewed and updated at a frequency that ensures that they remain fit for purpose.
i) Obsolete controlled documents are dated and marked as obsolete.
j) At least one copy of an obsolete controlled document is retained for a specified time period in accordance with applicable specified requirements.

REMARKS

Many of the requirements in 4.3 overlap with elements of Control of Records (4.13). If you are doing this for the first time, it is not uncommon to have documents spread all over the lab and in different places on your computer. To complicate things further, you may also have many versions of the same document. If so, your first step is to identify and collect all hard and soft documents. You may find that the version that is approved by the laboratory director is different from the version in the department supervisor's office and both of which are different than the version being used by the bench tech. This is exactly the situation that document control is designed to avoid. Having different versions of a procedure means that there is insufficient control of the process, which can cause confusion and affect the quality of the data you generate.

There is no easy way to tackle this problem except painstakingly searching file cabinets, drawers, shelves, and computer logs. This will require help and effort from everyone in the laboratory. It is useful to get agreement from everyone first. Some laboratory personnel may be reluctant to give up their treasured hard copies even if these documents are obsolete. You may find varied versions of documents in nontechnical areas as well, such as customer service, marketing, and administration. Therefore, a laboratory-wide effort is required.

Once you have collected your documents, take an inventory. We recommend you do NOT simply discard old documents because your document management system likely requires you to retain obsolete documents for a specified period of time. In saying this, however, once you have identified old documents that fall outside your document management protocol retention rules, you should consider discarding them. The fewer documents there are to control, the easier it is to control them.

After you have identified all current documents (and discarded documents when appropriate), now comes the task of creating a system that complies with the ISO 15189 standard as referenced above. There are a number of ways to do this, so work with your LEAP coach. LEAP coaches can help you understand your needs as well as help you build a system that best meets those needs (preferably using LEAP). LEAP is equipped with a comprehensive ISO 15189-compliant document management system, but there are other software products that can also help you manage documents. Note that, while other systems may accomplish similar things, they will vary in utility and effectiveness. The policies and procedures defined in LEAP are based on the assumption that you will manage your main documents on LEAP.

Remember that this standard applies to all documents that are required by the QMS. This includes external normative documents such as accrediting organization policies, accrediting organization standards (such as ISO 15189 or CAP standards), and package inserts (if used by procedures). While these do not need to be approved by the laboratory director, the laboratory must have some mechanism to control these documents and ensure that the lab has a method to update the version when the external source updates their version and that all relevant laboratory personnel have access to the current versions.

Please note that this FOS applies to all documents in all departments within the laboratory. You should aim to divide this detailed task with the appropriate department personnel but have a universal system that will apply to all sections (e.g., numbering of documents, version control). The documents themselves should be managed by each individual department or the Quality Assurance Department can be responsible for doing a periodic check of all documents within the laboratory to ensure that the documents are maintained using the universal system.

The best way to maintain your system is to make sure everyone in the laboratory is trained on how the document control system works and why it is important to keep everything up-to-date. Close attention to detail during audits is also important. Opportunities for training and improvement often come to light during audits. While there may be cases where you choose to use a paper-based system, the best way to become and remain compliant is to use LEAP for as much of your document management needs as possible. Even if you do not use all the features in LEAP, the MEF and MF folders can help you indicate the versions and locations of all your documents.

Periodic review of policies and procedures is important to ensure that they are current with standard practice and that the laboratory has not made any undocumented changes to procedures, instruments, systems, etc. Since different national or regional requirements may apply, ISO 15189 does not define the frequency of review. The laboratory is ultimately responsible for determining the frequency based on local requirements and the laboratory's needs. If the laboratory determines that the review is to be performed more frequently than required by local standards, auditors will require adherence to laboratory-defined periodicity.

Lastly, beware of brief procedure bench notes, posted short-cuts, instructions or "cheat-sheets". The reality is that people create bench notes to help them manage testing protocols. One of the biggest error labs make is changing the primary procedure manual while failing to change the "secret" bench notes. This may result in errors lasting years and can do real damage. Whether you accept bench notes or not is your decision. But, if you do treat bench notes in the same manner as other documents and manage version control, it is best to have them approved for use while ensuring they are cross-referenced to the applicable primary procedure manuals by including version identifications and appear in lists of controlled copies.

Why being in compliance with this FOS is important:

Failure to maintain adequate document control is one of the primary causes of error in the laboratory. Examples abound: biological ranges on patient reports, changes in software parameters, quality control shifts, and changes in policies and procedures can all lead to economic loss, increase in patient mortality and morbidity, and increased medical-legal risk. Your document management system is also the source for researching the root cause of errors, helping to identify possible quality indicators, and tracking the success or failure of implementing these quality indicators. A well-managed document management system is one of the hallmarks of a quality laboratory, allowing all the gears to turn smoothly and together.

As a reminder, laboratory quality should be aimed at reducing unwanted variability in test results. Without rigid control of documents, the laboratory risks introducing variability to its test results.

Materials Included In This FOS
• Document Control Policies and Procedures
• List of Controlled Documents
• Document Management Audit Checklist

FOS: Organization Responsibilities / ISO 4.1.1.1, 4.1.1.2

4.1.1 Organization

4.1.1.1 General

The medical laboratory (hereafter referred to as the laboratory) shall meet the requirements of this International Standard when carrying out work at its permanent facilities, or in associated or mobile facilities.

REMARKS

This article is aimed at clarifying that all protocols, procedures, and processes you enact as a result of becoming an ISO 15189 certified laboratory will remain in place in all facilities (mobile and permanent). This includes things such as External Drawing Stations and Point-of-Care Testing. You can insure constant compliance by setting up and monitoring all Processes using LEAP.

4.1.1.2 Legal Entity

The laboratory or the organization of which the laboratory is a part shall be an entity that can be held legally responsible for its activities.

REMARKS

You need to have a licensed facility that meets all local standards including staff with all legally required qualifications. This could mean your department of health regulations pertaining to the clinical laboratory, meeting local employment regulations, building codes, fire codes, infectious disease reporting requirements, and any other local laws or regulations. At a minimum, you will want to keep copies of all Medical Technologist (MT) licenses, Ph.D. diplomas, and M.D. diplomas. If MT licenses are not required, you must keep the education diplomas and transcripts to demonstrate that you meet required qualifications. While this may be a policy generated from the Laboratory Director Department, the actual documents may be maintained by the Personnel Department.

Note that if you use LEAP effectively, your staff will be unable to falsify document dates due to the embedded timestamps and further reflected in the timegraphs on the LEAP Maintenance Dashboard of each department.

Why being in compliance with this FOS is important:

If you do not follow ISO 15189 requirements, your laboratory may jeopardize its accreditation status. This could take you out of contractual compliance and hurt your reputation. Not complying with local regulations could bring fines, loss of funding, and—in some cases—even criminal prosecution.

We all know that it is possible to be in compliance at the time of inspection and out of compliance shortly thereafter. This method of maintaining accreditation or certification is not only a general waste of time and effort (i.e., you get all the costs and few of the benefits), it also corrupts your culture, making it ok to falsify document dates. When management gives implicit approval for these kinds of behaviors, this could lead to other similar behaviors such as with quality control and even patient data.

Of course, if you use LEAP, this kind of corrupting behavior is nearly impossible due to the ongoing tracking of QMS maintenance, exposing the issues at the point of inspection. LEAP will help you attain the goal of continuous compliance.

Materials Included In This FOS
• Organization Responsibilities Policies and Procedures
• List of Legal Requirements and Licenses, Permits, and Certificates Log Sheet

FOS: Management Responsibilities / ISO 4.1.1.3

4.1.1.3 Ethical Conduct

Laboratory management shall have arrangements in place to ensure the following:

a) There is no involvement in any activities that would diminish confidence in the laboratory's competence, impartiality, judgment or operational integrity;

REMARKS

To confirm if you are in compliance, you need to ask yourself questions such as: Are you favoring vendors because they are family or friends? Are you using reagents beyond their expiration dates and/or without validating their viability? Are you employing people unqualified for their jobs? Have your employees' competency been assessed? Are you paying all required taxes? Are you doing business with vendors without contracts?

b) Management and personnel are free from any undue commercial, financial or other pressures and influences that may adversely affect the quality of their work;

REMARKS

To confirm if you are in compliance, you need to ask yourself questions such as: Are you buying from vendors based on social or financial obligations or because the vendor offers the most preferable product or commercial terms? Is your budget so restricted that you are unable to perform Quality Control properly? Are there instances of nepotism within the organization that may impact quality? That is not to say that family members may not work in the same organization, only that these are recognized, openly declared (as noted below in c), and do not impact quality.

c) Where potential conflicts in competing interests may exist, they shall be openly and appropriately declared;

REMARKS

Conflicts and even conflicts of interest are a reality in any organization. These may be based on historical, personnel, or legal issues. If you have any of these kinds of conflicts or others, you need to officially identify the potential conflicts. Of course, we recommend that you work toward resolving these issues expediently; moreover, we recommend you do not try to hide or ignore these issues. Experience shows that covering up or ignoring conflicts inevitably leads to greater problems, typically in excess of the actual potential conflict. There is no prohibition on having conflicts of interest. These must just be openly declared.

d) There are appropriate procedures to ensure that staff treat human samples, tissues or remains according to relevant legal requirements;

REMARKS

While it is up to each laboratory to assess all laws and regulations and implement conforming procedures, a rule of thumb is that all biologic specimens be treated as if potentially infectious and could cause the transmission of disease. From harvesting to inventorying to discarding, we recommend that processes be put in place to best ensure that staff and/or the general public remain safe. This includes having biologic hazards properly identified and Personal Protective Equipment (PPE) be used in accordance with lab safety policies.

e) Confidentiality of information is maintained.

REMARKS

Given current privacy laws, maintaining confidentiality is of utmost importance. This can be handled through password protection of digital files, anonymization of patient data, and/or storage of physical files under lock-and-key.

Why being in compliance with this FOS is important:

There are a great many things that cause problems when a laboratory fails to have or comply with ethics policies. If you give favoritism to one vendor, it may mean that you are spending too much of your precious budget by decreasing competitive pressures. Not performing competency assessments or showing favoritism to one employee over another can degrade confidence in laboratory leadership and lead to unproductive behaviors. All of this can have detrimental effects on safety and ability to contribute to quality patient outcomes.

Having and adhering to an ethics policy can pay great dividends as it increases transparency, fosters staff morale, and projects a positive aura to patients and providers.

Materials Included In This FOS
• Management Responsibilities Policies and Procedures
• Ethics Policy

FOS: Management Commitment / ISO 4.1.2.1

It is recommended that the laboratory director delegates much of the work required to fulfill the management commitment responsibilities. These duties are typically delegated to the quality assurance and personnel managers. The laboratory director needs to review that all functions are performed and take appropriate action when necessary. These duties may only be delegated to individuals with the qualifications to perform those tasks. A director can delegate the performance of the task, but the laboratory director maintains responsibility that the tasks are done properly, and must have a process to a process to monitor the performance of those to whom he has delegated. Lastly, there are some duties that may not be delegated. All of these duties and delegations can be performed and recorded in LEAP.

4.1.2 Management Responsibility

4.1.2.1 Management Commitment

Laboratory management shall provide evidence of its commitment to the development and implantation of quality management system and continually improve its effectiveness by:

a) Communicating to laboratory personnel the importance of meeting the needs and requirements of users (see 4.1.2.2) as well as regulatory and accreditation requirements;

REMARKS

The easiest way to ensure your laboratory staff understands your laboratory's policies and regulatory requirements is to use the LEAP education and confirmation systems. You can also share the meeting minutes of QA meetings by adding the appropriate people as maintenance team members to the LEAP Maintenance Protocol.

b) Establishing the quality policy (see 4.1.2.3);

REMARKS

A sample Quality Policy is included in the FOS templates. Review this template and adapt it to the specific needs of your laboratory. Remember, your Quality Policy should be reviewed and modified, as appropriate, on a regular basis and included in your LEAP Maintenance Protocol. Make sure to relate your Quality Policy with your Quality Objectives. Note that your Quality Policy will be managed by the Quality Manager (refer to f) below).

c) Ensuring that quality objectives and planning are established (see 4.1.2.4);

REMARKS

A sample Quality Objectives is included in the FOS templates. Review this template and adapt it to the specific needs of your laboratory. You need to consider your Quality Policy when determining your specific Quality Objectives. LEAP will require your Quality Policy and Objectives to be reviewed and modified, as appropriate, on a regular basis. Note that, for ease of operation, LEAP has combined the Quality Policy and Objectives into a single template that will be managed under a single LEAP Maintenance Task.

d) Defining responsibilities, authorities and interrelationships of all personnel (see 4.1.2.5);

REMARKS

In larger labs, the defining of responsibilities, authorities, and interrelationships of all personnel is typically accomplished by using an Organizational Chart, related Job Descriptions, and a Delegation Chart. While the Organizational Chart will be managed in this FOS (as it should be one of the first matters you define), related Job Descriptions and Delegation Charts are included in the LEAP Personnel Department Laboratory Director Responsibilities FOS. The laboratory director needs to monitor this, but it is best if these documents are created and managed within the Personnel Department. The Organizational Chart should also include the relationship of the laboratory to the parent organization (if applicable, refer to 4.2.2.2 (c)).

e) Establishing communication processes (see 4.1.2.6);

REMARKS

The Organizational Chart can be used to define communication pathways for QA issues. Establishing communication processes is essential to a properly functioning laboratory and, if the Organizational Chart is insufficient, can be included within your Job Descriptions and Delegation Chart. You will need to consider both routine communications and emergency communication protocols. Also, emergency communication is typically needed in the case of patient-related emergencies or staff safety emergencies. A sample Communication Protocol is available in the FOS templates.

f) Appointing a quality manger, however named (see 4.1.2.7);

REMARKS

The laboratory must assign a qualified person to be in charge of overall laboratory quality. In the early days of your QMS journey, identifying such a person may be difficult. However, over time and with ongoing training and support, the appointed person will grow into the position. The key is to identify a person who has a good understanding of laboratory science and understands how the lab's organization functions. They will need to be willing to listen, study, and learn. The best candidate should have good communication and leadership skills and be respected by their peers. Remember your quality manager will be one of the most important people leading your laboratory along your QMS journey. Also, it is important that this person report directly to laboratory management or director. A quality manager who is beholden to a testing department or director cannot be effective in monitoring that department.

g) Conducting management reviews (see 4.15);

REMARKS

Management reviews need to occur on a regular basis and in accordance with the laboratory's policies and procedures. This is typically managed by the quality manager, and all records are maintained in the Quality Assurance Department.

The laboratory director should review these records saved within LEAP periodically and note any observations made during this review.

> h) Ensuring that all personnel are competent to perform their assigned activities (see 5.1.6);

REMARKS

Establishing and reviewing competency for all your employees is a vital job and perhaps a manager's most important task. This is typically managed by your Personnel Department Competency Assessment FOS but needs to be overseen by the laboratory director. This oversight can be recorded by commenting within LEAP.

> i) Ensuring availability of adequate resources (see 5.1, 5.2 and 5.3) to eneable the proper conduct of pre-examination, examination and post-examination activities (see 5.4, 5.5 and 5.6);

REMARKS

Determining if your laboratory has adequate resources to meet the needs of your users can be best performed by monitoring management reviews, internal audits and quality indicators. In case you determine needs are not being met, you should create a quality indicator and manage corrective within quality assurance meetings. You can also include an analysis that you have available resources as part of your evaluation of bringing new testing, changes in methodology or significant increases in test volume.

Why being in compliance with this FOS is important:

Assigning an independent quality manager, clearly defining your Organizational Chart and identifying details for related job descriptions for all personnel, as well as creating an overarching Quality Policy and Objectives will deliver a clear message to your staff and users about why you are going through the QMS process. Failure to do this effectively may result in people 'going through the motions' without an understanding of the ultimate goals, potentially creating ineffective systems. On the other hand, getting a motivated and clearly targeted quality manager who communicates the lab's Quality Policy and Objectives as a constant drumbeat can create a more collaborative and positive environment and become the foundation of your quality system and thereby greatly enhance safety and best support patient outcomes.

Materials Included In This FOS
• Management Commitment Policies and Procedures
• Quality Manager Appointment Letter
• Quality Policy and Quality Objectives
• Organization Chart
• Communication Protocol

FOS: Needs of Users / ISO 4.1.2.2, 4.1.2.5, 4.1.2.6

4.1.2.2 Needs of Users

Laboratory management shall ensure that laboratory services, including appropriate advisory and interpretive services, meet the needs of patients and those using the laboratory services (see also 4.4 and 4.14.3.)

REMARKS

You need to consider all aspects of testing when determining your compliance with appropriate advisory and interpretive services. Are your phlebotomists trained to answer questions from patients? Are there people available who can explain to clients the methodologies employed by the lab and why these methods were chosen? And, of course, the laboratory must have medical resources available to help clients with medical interpretation of laboratory results specific to individual cases. For these latter instances, it is ideal to have clinicians with laboratory training. In many cases, this may be the laboratory director or clinical consultant.

4.1.2.5 Responsibility, Authority and Interrelationships

Laboratory management shall ensure that responsibilities, authorities and interrelationships are defined, documented and communicated within the laboratory organization. This shall include the appointment of person(s) responsible for each laboratory function and appointment of deputies for key managerial and technical personnel.

NOTE: It is recognized that in smaller laboratories individuals can have more than one function and that it could be impractical to appoint deputies for every function.

REMARKS

This theme is found throughout this FOS and cascades down from the Organization Chart to Job Descriptions to Delegation Charts. 4.1.2.5 specifically relates to management delegation for primary and secondary routes of authority. What happens when the main clinical chemistry system goes down and there are urgent patient samples waiting but the supervisor is not available? What happens if the laboratory director is the person responsible for handling inquiries from clients, and an urgent matter comes from the ER and he/she is not available? You need to look throughout your lab's organization, understand these interrelationships, and plan for contingencies.

4.1.2.6 Communication

Laboratory management shall have an effective means for communicating with staff (see also 4.14.4). Records shall be kept of items discussed in communication meetings.

Laboratory management shall ensure that appropriate communication processes are established between the laboratory and its stakeholders and that communication takes place regarding the effectiveness of the laboratory's pre-examination, examination, and post-examination processes and quality management system.

REMARKS

Within a good QMS, key communication at all levels needs to be documented. The reasons for this are to avoid miscommunications and to provide a way of retrospectively troubleshooting problems so guidelines can be created for future situations. Staff communications can take the form of memos and/or meeting minutes, while communications with clients can be recorded by logging emails, complaint forms, inquiry logs, and phone logs. Communications with vendors can be in the form of meeting minutes, logging of emails, and even contracts can be used. The key to all of these communications is that they are documented either on paper or electronically and that they are catalogued in a way that allows searching. All participants need to be clearly identifiable and the date (and time, if appropriate) must be clear. The best communications are clear and concise. This must be included in your Document Control (see also ISO Requirement 4.3 / Laboratory Director Department FOS Document Control).

Why being in compliance with this FOS is important:

ISO principles are geared to fulfilling user needs which is the whole reason that the laboratory or any organization exists. There are numerous potential liabilities if you fail to adhere to Needs of Users Standards. Unqualified people answering questions can create errors. Someone can fail to respond appropriately and document inquiries which can lead to inefficiencies and potential lapses in patient care. If you fail to deliver the services that users need, dissatisfaction and the loss of customers can occur. The lack of clear communication lines is something else that can cause confusion, tardiness, inefficiencies, and mistakes. Alternatively, creating and maintaining the Needs of Users Standards effectively can increase efficacies and save time through the use of your FAQ system and through disclosing and resolving important issues at your QA and management review meetings. When everyone understands lines of authority and communication, the entire lab will probably run more smoothly.

Materials Included In This FOS
• Needs of Users Policies and Procedures
• Authorization List for Inquiry Correspondence
• Inquiry Log Sheet
• FAQ Sheet

FOS: Quality Indicators / ISO 4.14.7

Please note that the text noted in shaded boxes is the actual ISO **requirement**.

4.14.7 Quality Indicators

The laboratory shall establish quality indicators to monitor and evaluate performance throughout critical aspects of pre-examination, examination and post-examination processes.

EXAMPLE: Number of unacceptable samples, number of errors at registration and/or accession, number of corrected reports.

The process of monitoring quality indicators shall be planned, which includes establishing the objectives, methodology, interpretation, limits, action plan and duration of measurement.

The indicators shall be periodically reviewed, to ensure their continued appropriateness.

NOTE 1: Quality indicators to monitor non-examination procedures, such as laboratory safety and environment, completeness of equipment and personnel records, and effectiveness of the document control system may provide valuable management insights.

NOTE 2: The laboratory should establish quality indicators for systematically monitoring and evaluating the laboratory's contribution to patient care (see 4.12).

The laboratory, in consultation with the users, shall establish turnaround times for each of its examinations that reflect clinical needs. The laboratory shall periodically evaluate whether or not it is meeting the established turnaround times.

REMARKS

It's useful to think of creating and maintaining Quality Management Systems (QMS) as a cascade of events. First, you have a quality policy to provide overall guidance. The next step is to provide quality objectives describing specific areas of desired improvement. This stage is followed by one in which you create specific, quantifiable quality indicators to drive your objectives forward.

Your quality objectives and quality indicators are determined by evaluating these objectives and indicators both in terms of fixing problems and also in terms of improvement. Lastly, you must develop target values or performance thresholds for all of your quality indicators. Improvement can occur in several forms such as increases in productivity, safety, economic and—most of all—elevating how the laboratory's work can improve patient outcomes.

Once identified and set up, these improvement-projects need to be tracked and documented until deemed concluded. You must then introduce new objectives and indicators. Start out with something easy and achievable with obvious quality implications so your staff can easily grasp the concepts. Then you can increase their number and complexity over time. As a LEAP user you can use the LEAP maintenance functionality to track and document all your Quality Indicator projects.

You will note that there are FOSs for tracking quality improvement in the Laboratory Director Department and also in all technical departments. If you are new to QMS, it may not be practical to manage quality indicator projects in all your departments. We recommend that at a minimum you have at least three (3) quality indicator projects on-going in the Laboratory Director Department. As your expertise grows, you can start introducing Quality Indicators into other departments. These projects will need to be managed by the designated quality manager

If you need some hints on determining your initial quality indicators, look in the LEAP samples found in this FOS Content Library. Modify the performance thresholds to be specific to your laboratory and situation.

Why being in compliance with this FOS is important:

Areas of desired improvement and the decreasing of risks can only be actionable with a plan and actions. Not executing a quality indicator program will lead to not fixing known problems and not improving upon known areas. This will lead directly to errors and accidents. Executing an effective quality indicator program will drive specific actions that will decrease error, increase productivity, safety and patient outcomes. This is perhaps the most important aspect of your quality journey.

Materials Included In This FOS
• Quality Indicators Policies and Procedures
• Quality Indicators Worksheet

PERSONNEL

FOS: Laboratory Director Responsibilities / ISO 4.1.1.4

4.1.1.4 Laboratory Director

The laboratory director shall be directed by a person or persons with competence and delegated responsibility for the services provided.

The responsibilities of the laboratory director shall include professional, scientific, consultative or advisory, organizational, administrative and educational matters relevant to the services offered by the laboratory.

The laboratory director may delegate selected duties and/or responsibilities to qualified personnel; however, the laboratory director shall maintain the ultimate responsibility for the overall operation and administration of the laboratory.

The duties and responsibilities of the laboratory director shall be documented.

The laboratory director (or designates for the delegated duties) shall have the necessary competence, authority and resources in order to fulfill the requirements of this International Standard.

The laboratory director (or designate/s) shall:

a) Provide effective leadership of the medical laboratory service, including budget planning and financial management, in accordance with institutional assignment of such responsibilities;
b) Relate and function effectively with applicable accrediting and regulatory agencies, appropriate administrative officials, the healthcare community, and the patient population served, and providers of formal agreements, when required;
c) Ensure that there are appropriate numbers of staff with the required education, training and competence to provide medical laboratory services that meet the needs and requirements of the users;

d) Ensure the implementation of the quality policy;
e) Implement a safe laboratory environment in compliance with good practice and applicable requirements;
f) Serve as a contributing member of the medical staff for those facilities served, if applicable and appropriate;
g) Ensure the provision of clinical advice with respect to the choice of examination, use of the service and interpretation of examination results;
h) Select and monitor laboratory suppliers;
i) Select referral laboratories and monitor the quality of their service (see also 4.5)
j) Provide professional development programs for laboratory staff and opportunities to participate in scientific and other activities of professional laboratory organizations;
k) Define, implement and monitor standards of performance and quality improvement of the medical laboratory service or services;

NOTE: This may be done within the context of the various quality improvement committees of the parent organization, as appropriate, where applicable.

l) Monitor all work performed in the laboratory to determine that clinically relevant information is being generated;
m) Address any complaint, request or suggestion from staff and/or users of laboratory services (see also 4.8, 4.14.3 and 4.14.4);
n) Design and implement a contingency plan to ensure that essential services are available during emergency situations or other conditions when laboratory services are limited or unavailable;

NOTE: Contingency plans should be periodically tested.

o) Plan and direct research and development, where appropriate.

REMARKS

You will find a recurring theme within QMS programs relating to personnel. Are your personnel qualified? Do they have the knowledge and skills to do the job? Is the job clearly defined? Are there regular assessments to ensure your employees are performing up to the specifications of the job description? Do you have documentation to justify all of the above?

In the clinical laboratory, while everyone is important, the position with ultimate authority is the laboratory director. This person has final responsibility to ensure the laboratory is operated in accordance with technical, clinical, and—in many cases—economic objectives. The laboratory director is also responsible for the safety of the staff. In many settings, the laboratory director has an additional responsibility to act as the bridge between the laboratory and clinical staff. This could include ensuring clients have adequate knowledge about interpreting test data and thus help respond to clinical emergencies. If there are systemic deficiencies found in the laboratory, these may also be cited to the laboratory director for failing to oversee those functions.

Let's address each key question that covers this requirement separately:

1) **Do you have documented laboratory director qualification requirements?**

Examine the laboratory director's job description and reflect on this when determining the minimum qualifications this job requires. Education level? Areas of expertise? Technical laboratory experience? Clinical experience? Management training? Management experience? Leadership traits? Licensure or certification requirements?

A laboratory director's ability to do the job effectively relies heavily on the person's ability to manage people, to appropriately delegate, and to oversee tasks. Leadership skills should be considered when determining the best candidate for the laboratory director.

Being the laboratory director is a big and challenging position regardless of lab size, and there is rarely the perfect person or someone that has all the required skills. Maintaining all the necessary skills and knowledge is an ongoing process.

2) **Do you have a laboratory director job description?**

The laboratory should maintain an up-to-date laboratory director job description that covers all the points listed in the ISO Standards. A sample Laboratory Director Job Description is also available in the LEAP Content Library.

3) Do you have laboratory director delegation documentation?

It is impossible for a laboratory director to perform all tasks and responsibilities by themselves. In some cases, the director may not be working full-time in the lab. In other cases, the director may have primary duties in a clinic or be doing patient testing in anatomic pathology. Regardless, it is imperative that the laboratory director clearly defines and delegates appropriate responsibilities to qualified personnel in the lab. Furthermore, it is the laboratory director's responsibility to ensure that the people delegated clearly understand the duties expected of them and perform these duties appropriately.

There are many ways to ensure that delegated responsibilities are made clear. One way is to build delegated authority/responsibilities into each job description. Another is to create a delegation chart or policy. While it is not an ISO requirement to have a delegation chart, it is a good way to clearly communicate lines of authority. A sample Delegation Chart is available in the LEAP Content Library.

It is important to remember that, although a laboratory director may delegate his/her duties to qualified personnel, it is still the director's job to take primary responsibility for all actions and outcomes. Specifically, a director may delegate the performance of a task but not the responsibility for it. The bottom line: make sure people delegated are qualified for the job. Make sure they are trained, make sure they understand their responsibilities clearly, and make sure they are doing them properly.

4) Do you have a laboratory director contingency plan?

What happens if the laboratory director is unavailable? This is especially important in the case of a critical event such as a clinical emergency or accident. You need to look at the critical functions that are directly the responsibility of the laboratory director and ensure there are alternative plans. These contingencies could be assigning duties to a second-in-command in the laboratory, having these duties go to an on-call qualified physician, or co-opting one or more laboratory director(s) from neighboring laboratories through mutual agreements. A sample Contingency Plan is available in the LEAP Content Library.

5) **What do you do when the lab hires a new laboratory director?**

The departure of an existing laboratory director and the hiring of a new one can be one of the most stressful times for a laboratory. Does the new director share the same vision as the last? Do they have a different management style? How does the lab handle the review and re-approval of all laboratory policies and procedures? This often takes a while and the laboratory needs to develop a schedule for procedure review. A sample Policy for New Directorship is available in the LEAP Content Library.

Why being in compliance with this FOS is important:

Clearly defining the laboratory director's responsibilities and ensuring that the staff understands these responsibilities is imperative to fulfilling the lab's mission. Symptoms of lack of clarity of director responsibility can manifest in confusion among laboratory staff and poor communication between the laboratory and clinical staff. This can lead to poor workflow productivity, economic waste, safety problems, and can contribute to poor clinical outcomes.

Clearly defining laboratory director responsibilities creates a quality work environment for laboratory staff, a clear understanding of the director's role in dealing with both day-to-day issues as well as emergencies, advances economic efficiencies, and creates good lines of communication between the laboratory and clinical staff, helping create quality patient outcomes.

Materials Included In This FOS
• Laboratory Director Responsibilities Policies and Procedures
• Laboratory Director Qualifications and Job Description
• Laboratory Director Delegation Chart
• Emergency Contingency Plan
• Procedures for Changes in Laboratory Directorship

FOS: Quality Manager Responsibilities / ISO 4.1.2.7

4.1.2.7 Quality Manager

Laboratory management shall appoint a quality manager who shall have, irrespective of other responsibilities, delegated responsibility and authority that includes:

a) Ensuring that processes needed for the quality management system are established, implemented and maintained;
b) Reporting to laboratory management, at the level at which decisions are made on laboratory policy, objectives, and resources, on the performance of the quality management system and any need for improvement;
c) Ensuring the promotion of awareness of users' needs and requirements throughout the laboratory organization.

REMARKS

The quality manager is the key person for implementing and maintaining quality in the laboratory. This is an important position for your QMS journey. This job and the laboratory director's job are the only ones specifically mentioned by position in the management requirements. An individual with the right skills and experience can make gaining and maintaining certification easier and more productive. This manager can also be a driver for vastly improved patient outcomes, decreased accidents, and improved economic circumstances for the laboratory as well as the healthcare system.

The ideal quality manager must understand all aspects of lab operations and have good organizational and communication skills. Special training in QMS is highly recommended. This training can come via formal education, distance learning, self-learning, and/or seminars.

It is recommended that laboratory management provide the quality manager with ample opportunities for ongoing education. If you do not currently have an appropriate quality manager, have an eager person start by studying materials found within LEAP, especially the LEAP Education Materials in the Content Library.

The quality manager needs to be empowered to do the job. The quality manager should report directly to the laboratory director and have the authority to call regular quality meetings, or have time allocated from regular staff meetings to review quality issues. There should be clear lines of communication between section managers and the quality manager. A quality manager who reports to a particular department cannot be effective in surveying that department.

Why being in compliance with this FOS is important:

While the laboratory director has final responsibility, he/she needs strong, qualified people to delegate to. This is especially true for a quality manager. Having a focused, independent, and dedicated quality manager means quality meetings, management reviews, and internal audits get scheduled and managed appropriately and will be the difference between driving quality indicators to fruition or just going through the motions. Performing these duties faithfully will ensure a safer, more productive laboratory that maximizes its contribution to better patient outcomes. Failure to appoint and support the right person will likely lead to a lackluster QMS with few of the attendant benefits from all your hard work and the resources invested in QMS.

Materials Included In This FOS
• Quality Manager Responsibilities Policies and Procedures
• Quality Manager Qualifications and Job Description
• Quality Manager Delegation Chart

FOS: ISO Personnel / ISO 5.1, 5.1.1, 5.1.2, 5.1.3, 5.1.4

5.1 Personnel

5.1.1 General

The laboratory shall have a documented procedure for personnel management and maintain records for all personnel to indicate compliance with requirements.

REMARKS

If your laboratory has a personnel department or personnel liaison with a hospital or head office, it is best that these issues are managed at that level. Otherwise, 5.1.1, 5.1.2, 5.1.3 and 5.1.4 are likely best managed by the laboratory director appointing someone in the lab to maintain the appropriate records.

Know that, when preparing for an internal or external audit, the quality manager should be able to access all of these materials.

5.1.2 Personnel Qualifications

Laboratory management shall document personnel qualifications for each position. The qualifications shall reflect the appropriate education, training, experience, and demonstrated skills needed to the tasks performed.

The personnel making judgments with reference to examinations shall have the applicable theoretical and practical background and experience.

NOTE: Professional judgments can be expressed as opinions, interpretations, predictions, simulations, and models and values, and should be in accordance with national, regional, and local regulations and professional guidelines.

REMARKS

In the simplest terms, 5.1.2 asks this: are your people qualified to do their jobs, and, if so, prove it. There are many ways to accomplish this, but the basic elements of complying with this article means clearly defining job requirements and cross-referencing them with employees' qualifications and experience.

The most logical way of addressing this issue is to first define the overall function of the laboratory. The second step is dividing the functions by departments and then further segmenting them by position, and, lastly, to document this for each employee. The easiest way to represent this concept is with an organization chart and clearly defined job descriptions (see 5.1.3).

Make sure you take special care to understand all legal ramifications. Some positions may require, for example, a medical technologist license. This is especially so when interpretation is required. For example, if someone is screening cytology samples, they will require specialized cytotechnologist education and may require a license. Failure to comply with these kinds of laws will not only alert the ISO auditor, it can also get your laboratory into legal trouble.

In some cases, on-the-job training (OJT) under the supervision of a qualified and licensed professional may substitute for education requirements. Take care, however, that, if a person is assigned to a job based on OJT experience, a licensed staff member may still be required to oversee the tasks and take primary responsibility and should document review of the work performed by the person assigned to OJT.

5.1.3 Job Descriptions

The laboratory shall have job descriptions that describe responsibilities, authorities, and tasks for all personnel.

REMARKS

In laboratories with a stable and long-term employment history, it is easy to become complacent and lax in defining and reviewing job descriptions. When veteran staff members know what to do, lab operations may seem to function effortlessly. But, when you go through the process of creating job descriptions, you may likely find that things are not as harmonious as you think. Creating job descriptions will reveal much about your operations, and you will likely find problems.

Creating job descriptions is a valuable exercise and an absolute requirement, not just for successfully implementing QMS but for a smoothly functioning laboratory. Job descriptions are necessary for everyone in both technical and support functions as well as for the laboratory director and for housekeeping. Everyone needs a job description that accurately corresponds with the laboratory's organization chart, and the assigned duties to each personnel should correspond to the individual's competency and professional assessment.

The secret to job descriptions to have each one correspond with the relevant employee's personnel qualifications (see 5.1.2). When creating job descriptions, we recommend you review the CV of each employee. It is also important to look critically at both the job description and the CV. You may find people unqualified for their positions or who are lacking sufficient documentation to prove they meet the minimum requirements.

In the event that you find someone with insufficient documentation to qualify for their assigned job, you will need to obtain the required documentation, find another qualified person to perform that function, or find a way to make that person qualified. This can mean documented OJT under the supervision of a qualified staff member, additional external education, or even documented self-study.

Please understand, if there are legal certification requirements, such as the cytology example mentioned above, *you will have no choice* but to meet that certification requirement regardless of the competency of your personnel. *You will not be certified as an ISO15189-compliant laboratory if you have unqualified people doing jobs legally requiring certification. You are also at legal risk if you continue to allow these people to perform such jobs.* Most professional certification programs require ongoing education and—in some cases—testing for individuals to retain their certified status. You need to have systems in place to regularly monitor the certification status for those employees requiring certification by law or by laboratory policy. If a laboratory accepts samples from several jurisdictions, a certification or license in each may be required.

5.1.4 Personnel Introduction to Organizational Environment

The laboratory shall have a program to introduce new staff to the organization, the department, or area in which the person will work, the terms and conditions of employment, staff facilities, health and safety requirements (including fire and emergency), and occupational health services.

REMARKS

When new employees are introduced into the laboratory, it's important to undertake and document an onboarding process. This will include reviewing with the new hire your rules of employment, including an explanation of the organization chart, their job description, and the job descriptions of the people they work with, and, of course, the quality and safety manuals must also be covered. You can accomplish all of these tasks by creating a new employee handbook containing all the generic information. Alternatively, you can create a checklist of items that each new employee needs to review. Make sure you document each new employee's onboarding. We recommend you do so by having the new employee sign a relevant document. Remember, all of your SOPs, organization charts, and education programs should be uploaded and available within LEAP as a convenient way for new employees to become acquainted with your laboratory's operations.

Why being in compliance with this FOS is important:

In the end, nearly everything is about people. If your people are qualified, know what their job is, and they understand their job in relation to others, your lab will run smoother, more productively, and will best promote quality patient outcomes. I don't think it takes much imagination to figure out how a lab will function if the staff are unqualified and don't understand their jobs. It's a disaster waiting to happen.

Materials Included In This FOS
• ISO Personnel Policies and Procedures
• Personnel Policies and Procedures
• Qualifications and Job Descriptions Form
• New Employee Handbook

FOS: Personnel Records / ISO 5.1.9

5.1.9 Personnel Records

Records of the relevant educational and professional qualifications, training and experience, and assessments of competence of all personnel shall be maintained.

These records shall be readily available to relevant personnel and shall include but not be limited to:

a) Education and professional qualifications;
b) Copy of certification or license, when applicable;
c) Previous work experience;
d) Job descriptions;
e) Introduction of new staff to the laboratory environment;
f) Training in current job tasks;
g) Competency assessments;
h) Records of continuing education and achievements;
i) Reviews of staff performance;
j) Reports of accidents and exposure to occupational hazards;
k) Immunization status, when relevant to assigned duties.

NOTE: The records listed above are not required to be stored in the laboratory, but can be maintained in other specified locations, providing they remain accessible as needed.

REMARKS

This is one of the most important and yet most tedious parts of the ISO process. It is all about assigning the right person to manage this information and organizing it in a way that provides transparency to the people who need to have the information and security for privacy of individual information.

In the previous FOS ISO Personnel, you created a generic Qualifications and Job Description Form for each position within the laboratory. For this standard, you will need to customize these specific position templates for each employee that fulfills this job.

We suggest using the employee checklists that can be found within the Content Library as a reference to build a file containing all required documentation for each employee including all new employees. New employees will need to demonstrate that they have the appropriate skills and knowledge to perform their job functions safely and effectively.

All private documents should be password-protected, and the password should only be made available on a need-to-know basis. For example, the laboratory director, head of personnel, and, in some cases, the direct supervisor can have access to sensitive information. You may also need to make these available to auditors in some countries.

When determining what should be open or private and password-protected, the general rule is "need-to-know." This rule is not universal for all personnel documents. For example, technical supervisors need access to competency assessments but not necessarily to performance reviews. If, on the other hand, the technical supervisor is also the department head, they will need access to both performance reviews and competency assessments. This can all be managed by different passwords for each level of desired security.

We recommend that you keep the New Employee Checklist and Annual Employee Checklist templates within the LEAP MEF. The completed checklists for each employee should be password-protected and uploaded to the LEAP MEF or the storage location should be noted within the comments.

Please note that, while records should be filed and maintained within FOS Personnel Records, the procedures to do so should be according to the Personnel Policies and Procedures created in FOS ISO Personnel.

Why being in compliance with this FOS is important:

Remember, personnel records are not required by ISO simply to make your life difficult. Failure to keep personnel records can put your laboratory at legal risk and be a drain on your lab's productivity. On the positive side, a well-maintained set of personnel records will help create a transparent and accountable environment where everyone knows their role and the path forward. People clearly understanding their jobs, lines of communication, and having clarity on their bosses' perception of their performance, will be the foundation for ever-improving quality.

The majority of critical errors in the clinical laboratory affecting safety and patient outcomes can be directly attributed to human error. Personnel records are a critical check and balance designed to mitigate this risk for the laboratory and for the director, who remains responsible for his/her employees' actions.

Materials Included In This FOS
• Personnel Records Policies and Procedures
• New Employee Checklist
• Annual Employee Checklist

FOS: Competence Assessments & Performance Reviews / ISO 5.1.6, 5.1.7

5.1.6 Competence Assessment

Following appropriate training, the laboratory shall assess the competence of each person to perform assigned managerial or technical tasks according to established criteria. Reassessment shall take place at regular intervals. Retraining shall occur when necessary.

NOTE 1: Competence of laboratory staff can be assessed using any combination or all of the following approaches under the same conditions as the general working environment.

a) Direct observation of routine work processes and procedures, including all applicable safety practices;
b) Direct observation of equipment maintenance and function checks;
c) Monitoring the recording and reporting of examination results;
d) Review of work records;
e) Assessment of problem solving skills;
f) Examination of specially provided samples, such as previously examined samples, inter-laboratory comparison materials, or split samples.

NOTE 2: Competency assessment for professional judgement should be designed as specific and fit for purpose.

5.1.7 Reviews of Staff Performance

In addition to the assessment of technical competence, the laboratory shall ensure that reviews of staff performance consider the needs of the laboratory and of the individual in order to maintain or improve the quality of service given to the users and encourage productive working relationships.

NOTE: Staff performing reviews should receive appropriate training.

REMARKS

Simply put, competency assessments determine if an employee understands how a job should be done, and performance reviews establish whether the employee is actually putting this knowledge into action, following established policies, and doing a good job at it.

Many accrediting organizations and governmental organizations require assessing all six elements noted in Competence Assessment as part of testing.

We recommend that you use the Competency Assessment Worksheet and Performance Review Worksheet available in the Content Library as a reference and customize these worksheets to suit your laboratory's needs.

You can use LEAP to store and manage both the worksheets and the actual assessments/reviews. Ideally, the records would be stored as part of the Personnel Records, but if it is easier for you to store all competency assessments and performance reviews in one location, separate from other personnel records, the LEAP MEF for this FOS is a convenient location. All completed files should be password-protected with only relevant personnel having access to these passwords.

While assessments are required at six months after initial assessment, all subsequent assessments are annual. We have created a maintenance task to cover both cases, and the interval should be set accordingly.

The most effective way to implement a competency assessment and performance review is for both the manager and employee to complete the items individually prior to the meeting. This will allow you to focus on areas where your opinions differ and make the process most productive.

Why being in compliance with this FOS is important:

Competency assessments and performance reviews sometimes need to be delicately communicated to employees. It is an acquired skill, but once it becomes a shared habit, these processes will provide for an open, trusting working relationship. The employer will gain an understanding of the obstacles and challenges faced by their employees, and the employees will have an avenue for their voices to be heard. It will also be an opportunity to learn about personal issues that could affect work performance. Any staff suggestions should feed into the laboratory's process (4.14.4). Mostly, it allows the laboratory management to learn not only if the employees are doing their jobs well, but it also provides the opportunity for the employee to describe their vision about their future in the organization, and/or for the employer to try and match this vision with the needs of the organization.

Failure to perform real and effective performance reviews and competency assessments can lead to a culture of mediocracy and communication disconnects that can impact productivity, safety, and limit the ability of the laboratory to maximize its impact on quality patient outcomes.

LEAP Procedural NOTE:

Depending on the size and complexity of your laboratory, competence assessments and performance reviews can be managed centrally or at the department level. For this reason, FOS Competence Assessments & Performance Review (ISO Standard 5.1.6 and 5.1.7) can be found in the Personnel Department as well as each technical department. This allows you the option of customizing how you use FOS Competence Assessments & Performance Review:

Option 1) *You can decide to manage all the actual records in FOS ISO Personnel in the Personnel Department and use FOS Competence Assessments & Performance Reviews to centralize the documentation that is used.*

Option 2) *You can decide to save the actual records in FOS Competence Assessments & Performance Reviews centrally. In this case, you would N/A all FOS Competence Assessments & Performance Reviews for each technical department and manage the records within the Personnel Department.*

Option 3) *You can decide to save the actual records in FOS Competence Assessments & Performance Reviews in each respective department. In this case, you can either N/A the FOS Competence Assessments & Performance Reviews within* *the Personnel Department or designate this FOS for non-technical general departments (e.g., QA, IT, etc.).*

LEAP Procedural NOTE 2:

Two different Competency Assessment Worksheets and one Performance Review Worksheet have been provided in the Contents Library. You should determine what is the best format for your laboratory and use these for your new employee assessments and subsequent assessments/reviews. Depending on how you decide to store your records and templates, you must save the customized templates in the appropriate LEAP MEF.

Note that the New Employee Checklist in FOS Personnel Records includes an initial competency assessment, and the relevant worksheet should be used to fulfill this requirement.

Materials Included In This FOS
• Competency Assessments & Performance Reviews Policies and Procedures
• Competency Assessment Worksheet 1
• Competency Assessment Worksheet 2
• Performance Review Worksheet

EDUCATION

FOS: Training / ISO 5.1.5

5.1.5 Training

The laboratory shall provide training for all personnel which includes the following areas:

a) The quality management system;
b) Assigned work processes and procedures;
c) The applicable laboratory information system;
d) Health and safety, including the prevention or containment of the effects of adverse incidents;
e) Ethics;
f) Confidentiality of patient information.

Personnel that are undergoing training shall be supervised at all times. The effectiveness of the training program shall be periodically reviewed.

REMARKS

All of the training materials listed above should be created as you implement and manage LEAP. You can either choose to build specific training materials for 5.1.5 or gather all the relevant material from different FOSs including the SOPs that you create as well as the LEAP Education materials and place them in the LEAP MEF for this FOS.

We do recommend, however, that you create a log documenting all employees who have undergone the above-referenced required training and when that training was completed. We have provided a log template and sample for your reference and should be customized to suit your laboratory.

It is a big job to ensure all your laboratory staff members have been trained during your initial compliance fulfillment project, but it is of equal importance to ensure that new employees also receive this training. We suggest you accomplish this through your new employee orientation system and record the completion of this new employee training on the New Employee Checklist found in FOS Personnel Records of the Personnel Department.

Why being in compliance with this FOS is important:

Education and training is likely the most important thing you will do to drive quality. Education takes policies and procedures you may have created in a vacuum and makes them actionable. Until something is actionable and meaningful action is taken, there is no value. A well-implemented training program means the difference between an empty shell of QMS and something of great value, leading to productivity gains, higher standards of safety, and of course, better patient outcomes.

Materials Included In This FOS
• Training Policies and Procedures
• Training Confirmation Worksheet

FOS: Continuing Education / ISO 5.1.8

5.1.8 Continuing Education and Professional Development

A continuing education program shall be available to personnel who participate in managerial and technical processes. Personnel shall take part in continuing education. The effectiveness of the continuing education program shall be periodically reviewed. Personnel shall take part in regular professional development or other professional liaison activities.

REMARKS

With the advent of the Internet, continuing education has never been easier or cheaper with free and paid courses readily available. Also, please do not forget about the growing library of educational materials found within LEAP.

To maintain certification, a minimum number of continuing education hours are often required. You can also create your own policy regarding the minimum number of required hours. Typically, this is based on the position held and type of license or certification (if required). Your regional or national government may also set a minimum amount of continuing education.

Beyond Internet-based education, continuing education may be individually based or take the form of lunch speakers and/or professional meetings. Whenever you purchase a new instrument system, make sure you take advantage of manufacturer training programs. Regardless of how you continually educate your team, please ensure you document all steps in each staff member's personnel files.

Also don't forget that, in addition to time, education costs money. At budget time, we recommend you do your best to allocate funds for education. Costs can include travel, meeting fees, software programs, overtime for personnel covering for those taking education, and fees for guest speakers. To save money and get even more efficiency from your education budget, work together with neighboring labs or other laboratories in your laboratory system.

Last, but not least, remember that, as a LEAP user, you also have access to Minapsys software. If you would like to set up an administrator account, please contact CGI. By setting up an administrator account, you can utilize the benefits of Minapsys by inviting relevant personnel to participate in collaboration using interesting and challenging questions. We encourage you to be creative and use real-life problems revealed in the laboratory. Minapsys can promote independent thinking and learning among people while allowing for communication and solving problems together.

Why being in compliance with this FOS is important:

Technology, management systems, and underlying science are changing at breakneck speed. It is easy for both management and staff to get tangled in their day-to-day routine and stop learning. This can leave your laboratory using old technology, or even using current technology in appropriate ways. This can lead to lowered productivity and increase in medical errors thereby affecting quality of patient care. Alternatively, an active continuing education program can turn your laboratory into a vibrant place of learning and exploration.

Materials Included In This FOS
• Continuing Education Policies and Procedures
• Catalogue for Continuing Education Programs
• Continuing Education Worksheet

FACILITIES

FOS: Facilities Management / ISO 5.2, 5.2.1, 5.2.2, 5.2.3, 5.2.4

5.2 Accommodation and Environmental Conditions

5.2.1 General

The laboratory shall have space allocated for the performance of its work that is designed to ensure the quality, safety and efficacy of the service provided to the users and the health and safety of laboratory personnel, patients and visitors. The laboratory shall evaluate and determine the sufficiency and adequacy of the space allocated for the performance of the work. Where applicable, similar provisions shall be made for primary sample collection and examinations at sites other than the main laboratory premises, for example point-of-care testing (POCT) under the management of the laboratory.

REMARKS

In many jurisdictions, regulations dictate maximum occupancy for any given room. Know that occupancy limits are typically *not* calculated by room size but rather by the amount of available floor space. This means you must subtract the space taken up by lab benches, storage units, and equipment. Know too that, typically, there are also regulations dictating aisle widths.

Irrespective of local regulations, what is considered adequate space for performing lab functions is generally a judgment call. This may be well below the maximum occupancy set by regulation. Additionally, check each testing area for the activities that occur there. Does microbiology have enough space? Is the area around the chemistry analyzer sufficient for safe testing? As such, opinions may vary and this can be problematic during external certification audits. You need to look at each work area and ask yourself the following:

a) Is there enough space for people to work unencumbered by adjacent co-workers even during peak hours?

b) Is there enough space to lay out, in an organized fashion, all materials as set forth in all SOPs for that work area? This would typically mean reagents, samples, and instrumentation.
c) When workspaces are fully occupied, is there enough space for people to walk through aisles without disturbing work activities?
d) Does each department or testing area have enough space for the activities in that area?
e) Is there sufficient storage space such that new shipments of reagents or equipment do not occupy valuable real estate in the laboratory?

If you can reasonably answer "yes" to these questions, you will likely be okay from a space perspective.

Please know that space perception is highly dependent on how organized a laboratory is. Clutter is the laboratory's enemy: it occupies space, increases the opportunity for error and accidents, and creates a poor overall work environment. If your lab has been infected with the "clutter bug", the only solution is through training and good work habits. (Perhaps a quality indicator opportunity?) Clutter can include old equipment no longer needed, hardcopies of documents or books that are obsolete, or supplies not put away.

One proven method in some labs is implementing what is sometimes called the "X-Y rule". This simply means that staff are told to organize materials on the bench using the X-Y axis, avoiding odd angles. It may sound silly, but performing self-inspections on a regular basis and enforcing the X-Y rule can greatly increase your lab's organization and help manage space requirements.

5.2.2 Laboratory and Office Facilities

The laboratory and associated office facilities shall provide an environment suitable for the tasks to be undertaken, to ensure the following conditions are met:

a) Access to areas affecting the quality of examination is controlled. **NOTE:** Access control should take into consideration safety, confidentiality, quality and prevailing practices.
b) Medical information, patient samples, and laboratory resources are safeguarded from unauthorized access.

c) Facilities for examination allow for correct performance of examinations. These include, for example, energy sources, lighting, ventilation, noise, water, waste disposal and environment conditions.
d) Communication systems within the laboratory are appropriate to the size and complexity of the facility to ensure the efficient transfer of information.
e) Safety facilities and devices are provided and their functioning regularly verified.

EXAMPLE: Operation of emergency release, intercom and alarm systems for cold rooms and walk-in freezers; accessibility of emergency showers and eyewash, etc.

REMARKS

A clinical laboratory environment containing patient samples and/or chemicals is considered a "dirty area"—in other words, a place where exposure is possible to potentially dangerous pathogens and/or chemicals. People untrained in the proper use of personal protective equipment (PPE) or those who have not undertaken infection control training are at risk when entering a clinical laboratory. As such, you need to develop systems that limit entry only to those with proper training. It is important that you clearly delineate between outside or administrative areas and the clinical laboratory with its possible infectious areas.

To create this clear delineation, we recommend installing signage identifying boundaries between clean and dirty areas. We further recommend having suitable places readily available for lab coat storage. You also should consider maintaining a PPE inventory next to laboratory entranceways. Having biohazard-labeled trash containers for discarded PPE near exists is also a good idea. Common sense dictates that PPE should not be worn into clean areas. Common sense also dictates that lab coats and other PPE should not be taken into clean areas.

Other reasons for limiting entry to qualified people is to better ensure patient privacy and to decrease the probability of accidents caused by people in unfamiliar environments.

You will need to determine your own methods of limiting access. Access levels and deterrents will be determined by level of perceived risk. For example, if your lab has a door to a public thoroughfare, you should keep this door locked. If, on the other hand, lab access is only through an adjacent lab office, your methods may be limited to signage notifying people that they are moving into a potentially infectious area, and possibly notifying them of a PPE mandate for entry.

It is also important to ensure that personnel who work in dirty areas have sufficient secure storage for their personal effects in a clean area. A handbag stored in a nearby drawer may contain food or medication. Eating, gum chewing, or manipulation of contact lenses must not be done in dirty lab areas. Also, lab management must lead by example.

5.2.3 Storage Facilities

Storage space and conditions shall be provided that ensure the continuing integrity of sample materials, documents, equipment, reagents, consumables, records, results and any other items that could affect the quality of examination results. Clinical samples and materials used in examination processes shall be stored in a manner to prevent cross contamination. Storage and disposal facilities for dangerous materials shall be appropriate to the hazards of the materials and as specified by applicable requirements.

REMARKS

Storage includes closets, drawers, refrigerators, freezers, and rooms designated as storage. It also includes filing cabinets and areas for record storage. Most qualified lab inspectors will tell you that one true yardstick of a lab's quality is its storage methods. Aside from things being neat, clean, organized, and labeled, we recommend you take special care of the following:

a) Flammable materials should be stored in a fire-resistant area, particularly if these materials are in volumes sufficient to burn down the lab (more than one material measuring at least 1000 mL is a good rule of thumb). Maximums inside or outside storage cabinets may be regulated by local authorities.

b) Acids and bases must be stored in separate cabinets, or in such a manner that breakage would not mix the two. If you need to know why, you should consider taking a basic chemistry course. (Ka-Boom!)
c) Poisons and/or drugs should be locked up, and a log should be maintained detailing who has access and what gets removed and/or added.
d) All samples, reagents, and chemicals should be labeled. Labels should detail content and expiration dates. This includes waste containers, cleaning agents, and even water bottles.
e) Unexpired spill kits should be located nearby, with adequate signage and posted (document-controlled) instructions for use.

5.2.4 Staff Facilities

There shall be adequate access to washroom, to a supply of drinking water and to facilities for storage of personal protective equipment and clothing.

NOTE: When possible, the laboratory should provide space for staff activities such as meetings and quiet study and a rest area.

REMARKS

Facilities guidelines are typically mandated by local regulations and labor laws and are usually dependent on employee numbers and/or expected external people-load.

Handicap access is increasingly required in many jurisdictions, and, of course, is highly recommended for healthcare facilities. Handicap access must take into account door widths, wheelchair ramps, and restroom facilities equipped with enough space for wheelchairs. Sturdy handrails should also be installed.

PPE includes things like examination gloves, lab coats, masks, and eye protection. All PPE should be inventory-controlled and maintained. We recommend you consider flushing eye-washes and safety showers regularly and that this maintenance be documented. (Using stagnant microbe-contaminated water when flushing your eyes after an accident is not a nice experience!)

Adequate areas for the secure storage of personal effects is also important. Be aware if any personal items can affect testing. For example, plants that produce pollen may produce artifacts on glass slides if located in the cytology processing area.

We recommend you include the review and documentation of these requirements in your internal audit processes.

Why being in compliance with this FOS is important:

Maintaining an organized, well-managed, well-equipped facility will decrease accidents, increase work productivity, and limit mistakes. A well-maintained facility will also increase the status of the laboratory in the eyes of other medical staff and patients. Remember, this is one area that is not budget-restricted. All it takes is staff training and management oversight.

Materials Included In This FOS
• Facilities Management Policies and Procedures
• Facilities Management Checklist
• Security/Privacy Protection Policies
• Visitors Log
• Safety Policy
• Electrical Safety Checklist
• Temperature and Humidity Log
• Dangerous Materials Log
• PPE Checklist

FOS: Environmental Conditions / ISO 5.2.6

5.2.6 Maintenance and Environmental Conditions

Laboratory premises shall be maintained in a functional and reliable condition. Work areas shall be clean and well maintained. The laboratory shall monitor, control and record environmental conditions, as required by relevant specifications or where they may influence the quality of the sample, results, and/or the health of staff. Attention shall be paid to factors such as light, sterility, dust, noxious or hazardous fumes, electromagnetic interference, radiation, humidity, electrical supply, temperature, sound and vibration levels and workflow logistics, as appropriate to the activities concerned so that these do not invalidate the results or adversely affect the required quality of any examination.

There shall be effective separation between laboratory sections in which there are incompatible activities. Procedures shall be in place to prevent cross-contamination where examination procedures pose a hazard or where work could be affected or influenced by not being separated. The laboratory shall provide a quiet and uninterrupted work environment where it is needed.

NOTE: Examples of a quiet and uninterrupted work area include cytopathology screening, microscopic differentiation of blood cells and microorganisms, data analysis from sequencing reactions and review of molecular mutation results.

REMARKS

Clinical laboratories manage many activities involving large numbers of people, and lots and lots of "stuff." This is a recipe for chaos and clutter. For some labs, reducing clutter and disorganization may be your single greatest challenge. If you can fix this problem, it will help significantly with QMS. In larger labs, trying to manage QMS centrally can be overwhelming so 5.2.6 is also included in all departments separately. Of course, such conditions may not apply to non-offending departments.

Although a single, major cleaning may appear to freshly organize things, keeping things orderly and systematized over the long term is more difficult and requires behavioral changes. As you probably know, asking people to change is one of the most difficult tasks there is.

If your laboratory is like many others, it is probably a mess. Our first recommendation is disposing of unneeded "stuff". Secondly, decide what materials you seldom use and arrange proper storage. If you are still using paper documents and records, go to FOS Document Control in the Laboratory Director Department and work on this problem as well. Some laboratory members may want rigidly to retain paper copies as well as old and outdated materials. Not only does this add clutter, it may also hamper document control. Examine everything in the laboratory. Consider discarding anything that does not positively contribute to the testing, is not part of R&D, or is not required by regulatory authorities. Note that LEAP can be an excellent way of storing many of your documents digitally.

After minimizing the number of things you deal with through disposal and storage of lesser-used materials, now it's time to empty drawers, clean under cabinets, and mop behind refrigerators. There may well be expired reagents (which need to be discarded or clearly marked if used for training). Remember, many of these areas might be contaminated, so use PPE.

After your laboratory is freshly cleaned and organized, now comes the task of keeping it that way. As mentioned in 5.2.1, one method proven successful in some laboratories is to implement what has been referred to as the X-Y rule. This simply means that staff are instructed to organize materials on benches using a X-Y axis avoiding odd angles. It may sound silly, but performing self-inspections on a regular basis and enforcing the X-Y rule can greatly increase your lab's organization and help manage space. It is much easier if maintenance becomes part of a routine rather than a once-yearly cleaning right before an external audit.

Regular general order, along with frequent cleanliness inspections (posting the results in the laboratory for everyone to see), are ways to change behavior. Of course, these actions are separate from your internal auditing process, but if you feel you have problems in maintaining neatness and cleanliness, you should consider implementing more regular inspections—in extreme circumstances, you should even consider daily inspections. Significant staff re-training may be required to exterminate this clutter bug. Of all the quality activities, this can be one of the hardest. You can also decide to make cleanliness a quality indicator.

Finally, it is important to keep incompatible laboratory activities separate. Nowhere is this more important than in molecular testing. Separation of pre- and post-amplification areas, unidirectional workflow, and task-specific laboratory coats are all environmental controls that help prevent cross contamination.

Why being in compliance with this FOS is important:

A cluttered and disorganized workplace translates to a cluttered and disorganized mind, which translates into errors, which translates to harm.

Materials Included In This FOS
• Environmental Conditions Policies and Procedures
• Environmental Standards Checklist

FOS: Quality Indicators / ISO 4.14.7

4.14.7 Quality Indicators

The laboratory shall establish quality indicators to monitor and evaluate performance throughout critical aspects of pre-examination, examination and post-examination processes.

EXAMPLE: Number of unacceptable samples, number of errors at registration and/or accession, number of corrected reports.

The process of monitoring quality indicators shall be planned, which includes establishing the objectives, methodology, interpretation, limits, action plan and duration of measurement.

The indicators shall be periodically reviewed, to ensure their continued appropriateness.

NOTE 1: Quality indicators to monitor non-examination procedures, such as laboratory safety and environment, completeness of equipment and personnel records, and effectiveness of the document control system may provide valuable management insights.

NOTE 2: The laboratory should establish quality indicators for systematically monitoring and evaluating the laboratory's contribution to patient care (see 4.12).

The laboratory, in consultation with the users, shall establish turnaround times for each of its examinations that reflect clinical needs. The laboratory shall periodically evaluate whether or not it is meeting the established turnaround times.

REMARKS

In many cases, your most obvious areas of improvement are related to facilities. Therefore, these can be easy and obvious areas for creating, managing, and completing quality indicators and can be something as simple as: cleaning and organizing your laboratory; getting rid of all useless old materials that have accumulated; organizing all the electrical wires; removing clutter from eye wash stations; or painting walls that have been splashed with stains in anatomic pathology. Usually a simple walk through the lab allows people to identify several obvious candidates for becoming quality indicators.

It's useful to think of creating and maintaining Quality Management Systems (QMS) as a cascade of events. First, you have a Quality Policy to provide overall guidance. The next step is to provide Quality Objectives describing specific areas of desired improvement. This stage is followed by one in which you create specific, quantifiable Quality Indicators to drive your objectives forward.

Your Quality Objectives and Quality Indicators are determined by evaluating these Objectives and Indicators both in terms of fixing problems and also in terms of improvement. Lastly, you must develop target values or performance thresholds for all of your Quality Indicators. Improvement can occur in several forms such as increases in productivity, safety, economic and—most of all—elevating how the laboratory's work can improve patient outcomes.

Once identified and set up, these improvement-projects need to be tracked and documented until deemed concluded. You must then introduce new objectives and indicators. Start out with something easy and achievable with obvious quality implications so your staff can easily grasp the concepts. Then you can increase their number and complexity over time. As a LEAP user you can use the LEAP maintenance functionality to track and document all your Quality Indicator projects.

You will note that there are FOSs for tracking quality improvement in the Laboratory Director Department and also in all technical departments. If you are new to QMS, it may not be practical to manage quality indicator projects in all your departments. We recommend that at a minimum you have at least three (3) quality indicator projects on-going in the Laboratory Director Department. As your expertise grows, you can start introducing Quality Indicators into other departments. These projects will need to be managed by the designated quality manager.

If you need some hints on determining your initial quality indicators, look in the LEAP samples found in this FOS Content Library. Modify the performance thresholds to be specific to your laboratory and situation.

Why being in compliance with this FOS is important:

Your facilities are the vessel in which you work and how you provide value to the system. It is also the face you project to fellow healthcare professionals and patients. A well-run and organized facility will surely lead to better productivity and project confidence for your work. All facilities have areas in need of improvement and all require quality indicators.

Areas of desired improvement and the decreasing of risks can only be actionable with a plan and actions. Not executing a quality indicator program will lead to not fixing known problems and not improving upon known areas. This will lead directly to errors and accidents. Executing an effective quality indicator program will drive specific actions that will decrease error, increase productivity, safety and patient outcomes. This is perhaps the most important aspect of your quality journey.

Materials Included In This FOS
• Quality Indicators Policies and Procedures
• Quality Indicators Worksheet

FOS: Patient Sample Collection Facilities / ISO 5.2.5

5.2.5 Patient Sample Collection Facilities

Patient sample collection facilities shall have separate reception/waiting and collection areas. Consideration shall be given to the accommodation of patient privacy, comfort and needs (e.g., disabled access, toilet facility) and accommodation of appropriate accompanying person (e.g., guardian or interpreter) during collection.

Facilities at which patient sample collection procedures are performed (e.g., phlebotomy) shall enable the sample collection to be undertaken in a manner that does not invalidate the results or adversely affect the quality of the examination.

Sample collection facilities shall have and maintain appropriate first aid materials for both patient and staff needs.

NOTE: Some facilities may need equipment appropriate for resuscitation; local regulations may apply.

REMARKS

For some patients, sample collection can be a very traumatic experience, and you need to be prepared for a variety of problems ranging from fainting to violent outbursts or even heart attacks. Examine your sample collection area and ask yourself what can be done to create a more relaxing, ideal environment. Improvements can range from more friendly colors to comfortable chairs and/or toys for children.

Once you have created the best environment, the next step is decreasing the likelihood for adverse situations to occur and for mitigating them if they do. This preparation includes things like having a place for patients to lie down, availability of first aid kits, and even resuscitation equipment. Think about everything that could go wrong and understand that, given enough time, they will. Plan accordingly.

Ensure that specimen draw areas give patients sufficient privacy. Based on local regulations, banks of adjacent patient draw stations may not satisfy privacy needs. Even curtains between draw stations may be insufficient. The degree of necessary privacy will be driven by regulation and social customs.

Language barriers can also be a major cause of patient trauma. Obviously, it is impractical to have staff with all possible language abilities, but you need to consider having language-capable people pre-identified to act as interpreters, particularly if there is a concentration of certain languages in your area. If this is impossible, you could have printed cards with the local language on one side and a non-local language on the reverse to allow at least minimal levels of communication. Some jurisdictions may require the laboratory to provide accommodations for different languages and for the hearing impaired.

Why being in compliance with this FOS is important:

Your sample collection area is likely the only area patients (and even clients) will ever see. If you provide sample collection services to wards, please remember that you are not providing a service but also presenting an image of the laboratory and either building or eroding trust. In conclusion, patients are the users of laboratory services and fulfilling user needs is central to the ISO standard requirements.

The sample collection area is the laboratory area that most directly impacts patient care and is the most visible. Most patient surveys cite their treatment and perceived treatment collection sites. If there are inadequate facilities for the handicapped, they may be deprived of care. If you exacerbate a blood-drawing phobia, these patients may be less likely to seek care. A laboratory that is prepared for an emergency and acts accordingly during one can have an extremely positive impact.

Materials Included In This FOS
• Patient Sample Collection Facilities Policies and Procedures
• Sample Collection Facility Checklist

LABORATORY INFORMATION SYSTEMS

FOS: LIS (Laboratory Information Systems) / ISO 5.10, 5.10.1, 5.10.3

5.10 Laboratory Information Management

5.10.1 General

The laboratory shall have access to the data and information needed to provide a service which meets the needs and requirements of the user.

The laboratory shall have a documented procedure to ensure that the confidentiality of patient information is maintained at all times.

NOTE: In this International Standard, "information systems" includes management of data and information contained in both computer and non-computerized systems. Some of the requirements may be more applicable to computer systems than non-computerized systems. Computerized systems can include those integral to the functioning of laboratory equipment and stand-alone systems using generic software, such as word processing, spreadsheet and database applications that generate, collate, report, and archive patient information and reports.

5.10.3 Information System Management

The system(s) used for the collection, processing, recording, reporting, storage or retrieval of examination data and information shall be:

a) Validated by the supplier and verified for functioning by the laboratory before introduction, with any changes to the system authorized, documented and verified before implementation;

   NOTE: Validation and verification include, where applicable, the proper functioning of interfaces between the laboratory information system and other systems such as with laboratory instrumentation, hospital patient administration systems, and systems in primary care.

b) Documented, and the documentation, including that for day-to-day functioning of the system, readily available to authorized users;
c) Protected from unauthorized access;
d) Safeguarded against tampering or loss;
e) Operated in an environment that complies with supplier specifications or, in the case of non-computerized systems, provides conditions which safeguard the accuracy of manual recording and transcription;
f) Maintained in a manner that ensures the integrity of the data and information and includes the recording of system features and the appropriate immediate and corrective actions;
g) In compliance with national or international requirements regarding data protection.

The laboratory shall verify that the results of examination, associated information and comments are accurately reproduced, electronically and in hard copy where relevant, by the information systems external to the laboratory intended to directly receive the information (e.g., computer systems, fax machines, email, website, personal web devices). When a new examination or automated comments are implemented, the laboratory shall verify that the changes are accurately reproduced by the information systems external to the laboratory intended to directly receive information from the laboratory.

The laboratory shall have documented contingency plans to maintain in the event of failure or downtime in information systems that affect the laboratory's ability to provide service.

When the information system(s) are managed and maintained off-site or subcontracted to an alternative provider, laboratory management shall be responsible for ensuring that the provider or operators of the system complies with all applicable requirements of this International Standard.

REMARKS

Problems with your LIS (Laboratory Information Systems) tend not to be isolated one-off problems. Rather, they tend to be built into your systems. Complicating things further, these problems tend to be hidden, locked within computer code that gets encrypted and unencrypted. All of this means that problems can exist for a long time and potentially impact large numbers of events.

Your LIS also has people problems, usually related to transcription. In fact, some people believe that the majority of errors in laboratory testing originate in manual transcription. The harsh reality is that 100% of transcribers make mistakes. The key to managing this is monitoring, evaluation, and training. Also, examining laboratory practices and limiting unnecessary data entry can reduce a laboratory's exposure. Instrument interfaces, online order entry, and voice recognition software can all diminish the likelihood of transcription errors, but, remember, sadly a zero error rate is impossible.

Some of the most common problems found in LIS are mistakes in units and decimal placement. One wrong flick of a finger during data entry can impact countless patients. Monitoring units is vital to decreasing LIS related errors.

Errors in calculations can also produce large numbers of erroneous reports. Ensure those areas of the LIS that perform calculations are protected and that calculations are periodically verified. This can include protecting cells in spreadsheets if they are used in calculations.

Remember that the laboratory is responsible for the results generated by software, *not* the computer or software vendor. Given that few lab personnel are software engineers, the question becomes how to verify performance of software and hardware systems. Although, in reality, the laboratory is dependent on vendor information for software performance, the laboratory can and must confirm the output of these systems independent of outside IT specialists. Before enacting any system, we strongly recommend generating tests and actual reports with every possible data iteration you can think of and do this on a regular basis, particularly after any software or hardware upgrade.

The ready tools you have within LEAP include your LIS Maintenance Checklist, Validation Protocol and Checklist, External Data Check System, LIS Failure Contingency Plan, Patient Confidentiality Protocol, and Test Order Protocol. We encourage you to take these seriously to help avoid embarrassing and potentially tragic errors.

Why being in compliance with this FOS is important:

Erroneous data can impact the diagnosis and treatment of patients, thus increasing mortality and morbidity. Even if caught early, these kinds of errors can expose the laboratory to ridicule and even legal problems.

Materials Included In This FOS
• LIS (Laboratory Information Systems) Policies and Procedures
• LIS Validation Checklist
• Patient Confidentiality Protocol
• Test Order Protocol
• LIS ISO Compliance Maintenance Checklist
• External Data Check Form
• LIS Contingency Plan

FOS: Access to Information Systems / ISO 5.10.2

5.10.2 Authorities and Responsibilities

The laboratory shall ensure that the authorities and responsibilities for the management of the information system are defined, including the maintenance and modification to the information system(s) that may affect patient care.

The laboratory shall define the authorities and responsibilities of all personnel who use the system, in particular those who:

a) Access patient data information;
b) Enter patient data and examination results;
c) Change patient data or examination results;
d) Authorize the release of examination results and reports.

REMARKS

If your laboratory is using a modern LIS, you will be able to give individual permissions to limit the scope of one person's activities. These permissions, however, are only as good as the surrounding security protocols. To know if your system is secure or not, you need to ask yourself the following:

a) Do all users need a password to gain access?
b) Are there rules about not sharing passwords?
c) Are there rules requiring people to sign-off from their workstations when they are not present?
d) Do you regularly change passwords and do passwords have minimal requirements to prevent hacking?

Failing to enforce rules limiting access to appropriate personnel means that the laboratory is not in compliance with the standards of 5.10.2, and you may be compromising patient confidentiality and safety.

If using a paper-based system, your challenge is to maintain as few paper copies with patient information as possible, and ensuring only need-to-know people have access to these reports. This typically means filing paper reports in filing cabinets and controlling access to these reports using keys and/or combination locks.

For a paper-based system, if you are managing a smaller laboratory, access can be limited to specific individuals. If you are running a large, complex laboratory, it is typically only practical to control this information on a position-level basis. For example, access to patient data or changing of reported data can only be done by laboratory managers, quality managers, and/or technical supervisors.

Managing who can change data, regardless of whether the laboratory uses a paper-based system or an LIS without variable permission access, is challenging and very important and can only be managed through proper use and maintenance of paper logs. For the record, it is never okay to change QC data.

In addition to safeguarding data, the laboratory must safeguard the LIS. This is to protect the programs themselves from unauthorized changes and safeguard the hardware from accidental or intentional tampering, ensuring that the environment for the servers is secure, and maintain adequate environmental controls. You need to ask yourself the following:

a) Has the system been adequately tested and validated both initially and after major hardware or software changes?
b) Are all aspects of the maintenance and use of the LIS documented?
c) Are the servers in a physically secure location with limited access?
d) Are there adequate protections and firewalls from intrusion?
e) Does the lab have adequate policies to protect from malware?
f) Does the server room have adequate environmental controls?
g) Are backups being done appropriately with some portion stored off-site?
h) Is someone alerted in the event of hardware failure or issues?

Why being in compliance with this FOS is important:

There are many issues for concern when discussing accessing and editing patient data. The main three include: 1) accessing sensitive patient data and exposing this to others; 2) changing patient data incorrectly and reporting results; and 3) modifying, updating, or altering software systems in a manner that impacts reporting (i.e., changing test value units).

The consequences of doing this incorrectly can be dramatic: you might report inaccurate results; patients' lives can be negatively impacted by privacy lapses; and the laboratory can suffer legal liability.

Beware of unintended impacts of software updates. Sometimes changes to programs, hardware, or operating systems can cause problems in other areas. Ensure that you adequately test and validate any upgrades. This include having a validation plan and following it.

Materials Included In This FOS
• Access to Information Systems Policies and Procedures
• Access Limitation Log
• LIS Privacy Protocol
• Policy on Data Changes

FOS: Quality Indicators / ISO 4.14.7

4.14.7 Quality Indicators

The laboratory shall establish quality indicators to monitor and evaluate performance throughout critical aspects of pre-examination, examination and post-examination processes.

EXAMPLE: Number of unacceptable samples, number of errors at registration and/or accession, number of corrected reports.

The process of monitoring quality indicators shall be planned, which includes establishing the objectives, methodology, interpretation, limits, action plan and duration of measurement.

The indicators shall be periodically reviewed, to ensure their continued appropriateness.

NOTE 1: Quality indicators to monitor non-examination procedures, such as laboratory safety and environment, completeness of equipment and personnel records, and effectiveness of the document control system may provide valuable management insights.

NOTE 2: The laboratory should establish quality indicators for systematically monitoring and evaluating the laboratory's contribution to patient care (see 4.12).

The laboratory, in consultation with the users, shall establish turnaround times for each of its examinations that reflect clinical needs. The laboratory shall periodically evaluate whether or not it is meeting the established turnaround times.

REMARKS

Given the speed of change in information technology, you should have no problem identifying areas that require improvement. Areas to look at in the Information Systems Department should include: data input/output, data storage, ease of use, reporting, ease of data traceability. These are just some of the topics that need to be continually assessed. Think about auditing work areas to ensure passwords are not posted, audit downstream report transmission to ensure transmission of accurate results, and periodically audit calculated results to ensure they are accurate. In the end, your greatest limitation may be budgetary, so use quality indicators to proactively lobby for the budget you need.

It's useful to think of creating and maintaining Quality Management Systems (QMS) as a cascade of events. First, you have a quality policy to provide overall guidance. The next step is to provide quality objectives describing specific areas of desired improvement. This stage is followed by one in which you create specific, quantifiable quality indicators to drive your objectives forward.

Your quality objectives and quality indicators are determined by evaluating these objectives and indicators both in terms of fixing problems and also in terms of improvement. Lastly, you must develop target values or performance thresholds for all of your quality indicators. Improvement can occur in several forms such as increases in productivity, safety, economic and—most of all—elevating how the laboratory's work can improve patient outcomes.

Once identified and set up, these improvement-projects need to be tracked and documented until deemed concluded. You must then introduce new objectives and indicators. Start out with something easy and achievable with obvious quality implications so your staff can easily grasp the concepts. Then you can increase their number and complexity over time. As a LEAP user you can use the LEAP maintenance functionality to track and document all your Quality Indicator projects.

You will note that there are FOSs for tracking quality improvement in the Laboratory Director Department and also in all technical departments. If you are new to QMS, it may not be practical to manage quality indicator projects in all your departments. We recommend that at a minimum you have at least three (3) quality indicator projects ongoing in the Laboratory Director Department. As your expertise grows, you can start introducing quality indicators into other departments. These projects will need to be managed by the designated quality manager.

If you need some hints on determining your initial quality indicators, look in the LEAP samples found in this FOS Content Library. Modify the performance thresholds to be specific to your laboratory and situation.

Why being in compliance with this FOS is important:

As a laboratory, the product you deliver is information. The faster, more accurate, more complete, and more flexible this information, the better results in the value delivered to the healthcare system and the greater impact on patient outcomes. Seeking out, defining, and driving excellence is exactly what Quality Indicators are designed to do.

Areas of desired improvement and the decreasing of risks can only be actionable with a plan and actions. Not executing a quality indicator program will lead to not fixing known problems and not improving upon known areas. This will lead directly to errors and accidents. Executing an effective quality indicator program will drive specific actions that will decrease error, increase productivity, safety and patient outcomes. This is perhaps the most important aspect of your quality journey.

Materials Included In This FOS
• Quality Indicators Policies and Procedures
• Quality Indicators Worksheet

SAMPLE COLLECTION

FOS: Sample Collection / ISO 5.4.4, 5.4.4.1, 5.4.4.2, 5.4.4.3

5.4.4 Primary Sample Collection and Handling

5.4.4.1 General

The laboratory shall have documented procedures for the proper collection and handling of primary samples. The documented procedures shall be available to those responsible for primary sample collection whether or not the collectors are laboratory staff.

Where the user requires deviations and exclusions from, or additions to, the documented collection procedure, these shall be recorded and included in all documents containing examination results and shall be communicated to the appropriate personnel.

NOTE 1: All procedures carried out on a patient need the informed consent of the patient. For most routine laboratory procedures, consent can be inferred when the patient presents himself or herself at a laboratory with a request form and willingly submits the usual collecting procedure, for example venipuncture. Patients in a hospital should normally be given the opportunity to refuse.

Special procedures, including more invasive procedures, or those with an increased risk of complications will need a more detailed explanation and, in some cases, written consent.

In emergency situations, consent might not be possible; under these circumstances, it is acceptable to carry out necessary procedures, provided they are in the patients' best interest.

NOTE 2: Adequate privacy during reception and sampling should be available and appropriate to the type of information being requested and primary sample being collected.

REMARKS

Sample collection includes, but is not limited to: venipuncture, urine collection, CSF, gross biopsy, dermatologic biopsy, needle biopsy, saliva, hair, feces, and sputum. Each of these requires its own collection procedure, complication risk profile, and inadequate sampling risk profile. Let's discuss several of these examples below.

Gross biopsy is typically a surgical procedure, but the anatomic laboratory needs to be involved in designing sample requirements. These include tissue-specific margin measurement and labeling requirements, minimum sample size, and container and preservative requirements. Referral surgical specimens should come with an original complete report. For frozen sections, maximum turnaround times need to be clearly defined and monitored. Patient consent needs to be included on the surgical consent form.

The needle biopsy procedure is performed in clinical settings. The collection method is technique-dependent and the collection risk profile is considered high. It is strongly recommended that patients sigh a consent form clearly delineating the risks. For cases of uteral needle biopsy, the consent form needs to include a clause indicating possible injury or death of the fetus. This consent form will typically be issued at the clinical level, but a quality laboratory may want to confirm that these consent forms are appropriate and completed prior to the procedure.

Cervical PAP smears are one of the most common laboratory procedures. Collection techniques are determined and performed by the medical facility. Regardless, it is the cytology laboratory's responsibility to ensure the adequacy of the testing sample. Patient and client information should be provided detailing the impact on assay sensitivity in case of a poor sample collection. We suggest laboratories consider recommending liquid-based cytology (LBC) methods because they are fast becoming the global standard.

Clear instructions and explanations as to why these above recommendations need following should be included when facilitating urine and fecal collection. Consent forms are not required by most laboratories.

If you are collecting sputum for lung cancer screening, patients need to know that test sensitivity is highly dependent on specimen quality and clear instructions are essential. While many labs use verbal explanations, you should consider a consent examination. Similar instructions need to be given when collecting microbial sputum for examination. (We also highly recommend a gram stain be performed on all sputum samples to confirm the presence of oral versus bronchial cell population. This is not, however, a specific ISO requirement.)

Venipuncture can be a traumatic experience for some patients. It can also have higher risk profiles for very young, elderly, and/or obese patients, as well as those with bleeding disorders. Losing consciousness is not uncommon. With a normal patient population, it is common practice to verbally explain the procedure and risks. With higher risk patients, however, getting an informed consent signed may be sensible.

Arterial puncture for blood gasses has its own unique risks. It is important that the patient understands these and the phlebotomist is trained to avoid them.

A comprehensive discussion on primary sample collection is beyond the scope of this document, but you can find more information in the LEAP Content Library.

5.4.4.2 Instructions for Pre-collection Activities

The laboratory's instructions for pre-collection activities shall include the following:

a) Completion of the request form or electronic request;
b) Preparation of the patient (e.g., instructions to caregivers, phlebotomists, sample collectors and patients);
c) Type and amount of the primary sample to be collected with descriptions of the primary sample containers and any necessary additives;
d) Special timing of collection, where needed;
e) Clinical information relevant to or affecting sample collection, examination performance or results interpretation (e.g., history of administration of drugs).

REMARKS

For venipuncture, it is important that the laboratory knows when patients are on any therapeutic agent for bleeding disorders including aspirin therapy.

You may also want to consider a special collection process for young children, neonates, elderly patients, and patients with diminished mental capacity. This may include purchasing and inventorying special collection devices and equipment.

Timing of collection can also play an important role for fasting glucose, lipid testing, and therapeutic drug monitoring. Clear instructions and protocols need to be created for collection site preparation.

5.4.4.3 Instruction for Collection Activities

The laboratory's instructions for collection shall include the following:

a) Determination of the identity of the patient from whom a primary sample is collected;
b) Verification that the patient meets pre-examination requirements [e.g., fasting status, medication status (time of last dose, cessation), sample collection at predetermined time or time intervals, etc.];
c) Instructions for collection of primary blood and non-blood samples, with descriptions of the primary sample containers and any necessary additives;
d) In situations where the primary sample is collected as part of clinical practice, information and instructions regarding primary sample containers, any necessary additives and necessary processing and sample transport conditions shall be determined and communicated to the appropriate staff;
e) Instructions for labeling of primary samples in a manner that provides an unequivocal link with the patients from whom they are collected;
f) Recording of the identity of the person collecting the primary sample and the collection date, and, when needed, recording of the collection time;
g) Instructions for proper storage conditions before collected samples are delivered to the laboratory;

h) Safe disposal of materials used in the collection.

Why being in compliance with this FOS is important:

There is risk involved in nearly all specimen sampling procedures. Not only does the laboratory need to minimize these risks, they also need to weigh these risks versus the clinical benefit. And, don't forget the risk to staff. The dangers of dealing with sharps together with biohazards should not be underestimated, particularly in emergency situations or with uncooperative patients.

There are really two main issues: equipment and training. Make sure you have the right tools for the job and make sure your people are proficient in their use. If you do this, risk will decrease and benefits will be more pronounced.

Materials Included In This FOS
• Sample Collection Policies and Procedures
• Sample Collection Manual
• Informed Consent Form

FOS: Pre-examination Processes / ISO 5.4, 5.4.1, 5.4.2

5.4 Pre-examination Processes

5.4.1 General

The laboratory shall have documented procedures and information for pre-examination activities to ensure the validity of the results of examinations.

REMARKS

Here are our goals for the following series of articles: to ensure that samples are collected in accordance with your SOPs; that clients and patients understand and are informed about details of procedures; that the laboratory collects the information you need to test and report results; and that you have a method to ensure that all samples can be traced to the patient. Creating and managing these systems is integral to any laboratory compliant with QMS and an important aspect to ensuring quality patient care.

While there are many ways to achieve quality patient care, the following materials will need to be created as you move through this part of your quality journey:

a) Laboratory Guide for Patients and Users
b) A system for collecting necessary information on each sample and patient
c) Methods for ensuring proper sample collection and handling
d) Sample transportation quality assurance procedures
e) Methods for receiving and storing samples

5.4.2 Information for Patients and Users

The laboratory shall have information available for patients and users of the laboratory services. The information shall include as appropriate:

a) The location of your laboratory;
b) Types of clinical services offered by the laboratory including examinations referred to other laboratories;

c) Opening hours of the laboratory;
d) The examinations offered by the laboratory including, as appropriate, information concerning samples required, primary sample volumes, special precautions, turnaround time, (which may also be provided in general categories or for groups of examinations), biological reference intervals, and clinical decision values;
e) Instructions for completion of the request form;
f) Instructions for preparation of the patient;
g) Instructions for patient-collected samples;
h) Instructions for transportation of samples, including any special handling needs;
i) Any requirements for patient consent (e.g., consent to disclose clinical information and family history to relevant healthcare professionals, where referral is needed);
j) The laboratory's criteria for accepting and rejecting samples;
k) A list of factors know to significantly affect the performance of the examination or the interpretation of the results;
l) Availability of clinical advice on ordering of examinations and on interpretation of examination results;
m) The laboratory's policy on protection of personal information;
n) The laboratory's complaint procedure.

The laboratory shall have information available for patients and users that includes an explanation of the clinical procedure to be performed to enable informed consent. Importance of provision of patient and family information, where relevant (e.g., for interpreting genetic examination results), shall be explained to the patient and user.

REMARKS

What you need to ask yourself is: what information will clients and/or patients need to know so they can be active and informed participants in the testing process? There are several ways you can accomplish this including: a) creating and maintaining a patient and/or client laboratory guide; and b) creating and maintaining a patient and/or client laboratory website.

Websites have several advantages. First is the ability to easily and quickly make changes such as adding or removing testing from your offerings and/or changing assay protocols. On the downside, some patients may not have access to the Internet—a problem solvable with print-on-demand for patients and clients who request paper copies. The most comprehensive solution is to have both a paper guide and website.

Why being in compliance with this FOS is important:

The laboratory cannot satisfy its mission alone. It needs cooperation and coordination from both patients and clinicians. From the clinicians' side, a lack of communication can result in improper sampling, improper labeling, improper transportation, inappropriate testing, and incorrect test interpretation. From the patients' side, failure to communicate can yield incorrect patient-derived histories or failure to prepare for testing, such as fasting requirements.

Materials Included In This FOS
• Pre-examination Processes Policies and Procedures
• Laboratory Test Guide
• Test Menu Specifications

FOS: Required Patient Information / ISO 5.4.3

5.4.3 Request Form Information

The request form or an electronic equivalent shall allow space for the inclusion of, but not limited to, the following:

a) Patient identification, including gender, date of birth, and the location/contact details of the patient, and a unique identifier;

   NOTE: Unique identification includes an alpha and/or numeric identifier such as a hospital number or personal health number.

b) Name or other unique identifier of clinician, healthcare provider, or other person legally authorized to request examinations or use medical information, together with the destination for the report and contact details;
c) Type of primary sample and, where relevant, the anatomic site of origin;
d) Examinations requested;
e) Clinically relevant information about the patient and the request for examination performance and result interpretation purposes;

   NOTE: Information needed for examination performance and results interpretation may include the patient's ancestry, family history, travel and exposure history, communicable diseases, and other clinically relevant information. Financial information for billing purposes, financial audit, resource management and utilization reviews may also be collected. The patient should be aware of the information collected and the purpose for which it is collected.

f) Date and, where relevant, time of primary sample collection;
g) Date and time of sample receipt.

NOTE: The format of the request form (e.g., electronic or paper) and the manner in which requests are to be communicated to the laboratory should be determined in discussion with the users of laboratory services.

The laboratory shall have a documented procedure concerning verbal requests for examinations that includes providing confirmation by request form or electronic equivalent within a given time.

The laboratory shall be willing to cooperate with users or their representatives in clarifying the user's request.

REMARKS

The objective of 5.4.3 is to ensure you have all the information your lab needs to collect the correct specimens, perform testing, report results, respond to enquiries, and proactively respond to problems impacting patient care and quality. The following are examples illustrating the importance of collecting data relating to your patients, samples, and clients:

a) A patient is on heparin therapy but this fact went unreported. When running a COAG panel, the technologist triggers a panic value and wakes the doctor in the middle of the night. The doctor is unhappy.
b) The only identifier for a sample is the patient's name. This name is very common, however, and the same batch has three identical names. A QC problem triggers a rerun for all samples, but the sample tubes were not placed in the right order, and there is no way to know which sample belongs to whom. The lab requests that all three samples be redrawn but only one patient is hospitalized. It takes two weeks to locate and redraw samples from the remaining two outpatients.
c) A sample shows a slightly elevated B-HCG level, but the patient's gender (male) was not listed. Also, unavailable to the lab is information that the patient was treated for testicular cancer three years prior. The results are reported on a routine basis, but the patient was on an overseas business trip and will not return for a month. Treatment for relapsed testicular cancer has just been delayed.
d) You get a call at 3AM from a client requesting that you add Gentamycin to the Test Requisition Form. The test is run and reported but the information is not placed on the Requisition Form so no charge was issued, resulting in a financial loss.
e) You are running a STAT 5 part differential on an emergency room patient. The results come back abnormal and are reported as such. Although the

patient has just returned from Thailand and has a high fever, none of this information was included on the Test Requisition Form. If the lab had known this information, the lab would probably have performed a blood smear immediately and reported it positive for malaria. The diagnosis and corresponding treatment are delayed.

Collecting comprehensive and accurate information on each sample and each patient is vital. Doing so brings the laboratory into the patient care loop in a comprehensive way, allowing you to actively participate in helping secure quality patient outcomes, increase productivity, and—in some cases—help the entire healthcare system save money.

Making a Test Requisition Form is the easy part. Making sure users fill out the form correctly is the hard part and takes leadership and effective communication from the laboratory to the clinical staff. Communication and feedback (both positive and negative) are key.

In some instances, it may be permissible to have a single patient identifier. Some clinical studies require only a patient code or study number to be used. Some testing may require anonymity. In these cases, it is vitally important that the laboratory and clinician have a mechanism to positively identify all samples.

Why being in compliance with this FOS is important:

Incomplete or inaccurate testing requisitions are a common and correctable cause of medical errors. In a busy medical practice, complete information allows the laboratory the opportunity to act as a back-stop for missing critical diagnostic indicators in support of the clinical staff. Moreover, a clear, easy to complete test requisition form and clear instructions communicated to the clinical staff can act as a vital information conduit between the lab and its users.

NOTE: *Do NOT accept and run unlabeled specimens. If the lab gets into the habit of running unacceptable specimens, you will encourage lax behavior in your clients. While users can be shocked by you rejecting unacceptable specimens, and you may feel obliged to accept these samples to avoid confrontation, it is much better for their patients in the long run if you strictly adhere to your rejection criteria.*

Materials Included In This FOS
• Required Patient Information Policies and Procedures
• Test Requisition Form

FOS: Specimen Transportation, Reception & Handling / ISO 5.4.5, 5.4.6, 5.4.7

5.4.5 Sample Transportation

The laboratory's instructions for post-collection activities shall include packaging of samples for transportation.

The laboratory shall have a documented procedure for monitoring the transportation of samples to ensure they are transported:

a) Within a time frame appropriate to the nature of the requested examinations and the laboratory discipline concerned;
b) Within a temperature interval specified for sample collection and handling and with the designated preservatives to ensure the integrity of the samples;
c) In a manner that ensures the integrity of the sample and the safety for the carrier, the general public and the receiving laboratory, in compliance with established requirements.

NOTE: A laboratory which is not involved in primary sample collection and transportation is considered to have satisfied clause 5.4.5 c) above when, upon receipt of a sample whose integrity was compromised or which could have jeopardized the safety of the carrier or general public, the sender is contacted immediately and informed about measures to be taken to eliminate recurrence.

REMARKS

While interpretation may vary, we should consider the issue of sample transportation in the following circumstances:

a) Transportation from hospital wards to a hospital laboratory
b) Transportation from a hospital laboratory to a referral laboratory
c) Transportation from an external drawing station or clinic to a hospital or referral laboratory

In each of the above circumstances, the risk of exceeding time and environmental limits varies. Also, the risk of accidental exposure increases the more a sample changes hands. Other variables affecting accidental exposure risk are the training of those handling specimens and the design of the logistics chain.

As risks increase, you will also need to proactively improve your prevention measures. Let's take, for example, the logistics of transporting a sample from a patient ward to the hospital lab. The main risk may be someone or something accidentally bumping into the sample cart. Therefore, you may have to consider protecting samples inside secondary sealed containers. At the other end of the chain, you may be using a third party freight vendor to send samples to an external referral lab. In this case, you may want to carefully evaluate the sturdiness of the primary container as well as use a secondary containment package that carries labeling identifying the package as biohazardous with instructions outlining what to do if leakage occurs.

When transporting specimens with higher risk factors for transmitting disease (such as suspected H1N2 or TB sputum samples), extra precautions should be considered. Potential strategies include special packaging, labeling, and the use of specialist delivery vendors.

Time is another important factor: time of sampling, shipping time, and time of receipt by the testing lab must also be considered if using outside delivery services. This information must be verified and documented in accordance with your established timing requirements. Similar systems should be considered for internal hospital testing environments. Methods include using time stamps on sample containers or employing HIS and/or LIS systems, if available.

Lastly, transport environments can be very important to specimen integrity. Does the sample need to be shipped at room temperature, refrigerated, or frozen? Have you supplied your clinic with the correct transport containers to ensure transport at proper temperature? For room temperature transport, do you need extra insulation during summer or winter months?

5.4.6 Sample Reception

The laboratory's procedure for sample reception shall ensure that the following conditions are met:

a) Samples are unequivocally traceable, by request and labeling, to an identified patient or site;
b) Laboratory-developed and documented criteria for acceptance or rejection of samples are applied;
c) Where there are problems with patient or sample identification, sample instability due to delay in transport or inappropriate container(s), insufficient sample volume, or when the sample is clinically critical or irreplaceable and the laboratory chooses to process the sample, the final report shall indicate the nature of the problem and, where applicable, that caution is required when interpreting the result;
d) All samples received are recorded in an accession book, worksheet, or computer or other comparable system. The date and time of receipt and/or registration of samples shall be recorded. Whenever possible, the identity of the person receiving the sample shall also be recorded;
e) Authorized personnel shall evaluate received samples to ensure that they meet the acceptance criteria relevant for the requested examination(s);
f) Where relevant, there shall be instructions for the receipt, labeling, processing, and reporting of samples specifically marked as urgent. The instructions shall include details of any special labeling of the request form and sample, the mechanism of transfer of the sample to the examination area of the laboratory, any rapid processing mode to be used, and any special reporting criteria to be followed.

All portions of the primary sample shall be unequivocally traceable to the original primary sample.

REMARKS

Sample reception and how your organization handles the process is usually a very accurate indicator of the overall efficiency of your laboratory. As such, it is an excellent opportunity to identify (and fix) problems and improve your lab's overall quality. As samples come into the laboratory, you need to ask the following questions for each and all samples:

a) Is the sample marked as "Urgent" or "STAT"?
b) Is the sample clearly labeled?

c) Is the sample container and preservative/pre-treatment appropriate?
d) What time was the sample collected and is it still within the time limitations for testing?
e) Is the sample volume adequate for testing?
f) Does the sample exhibit excess lipemia, hemolysis, or other visual abnormalities?
g) Is the sample within temperature specifications?
h) Does the sample display any evidence of leakage or tampering?
i) Is the transport tube or media expired?

Of all of these factors, the highest priority must be the urgency of the sample. We recommend that all urgent samples be handled under expedited conditions within the laboratory and are treated as urgent workflow as soon as identified.

Inevitably, you are going to receive samples that are unlabeled either because this step was overlooked or the label fell off. It may be possible to use the test requisition files to identify the case by a process of elimination. This is highly undesirable for many reasons. We recommend that all unlabeled specimens be rejected and recollected unless there are extraordinary circumstances (such as brain biopsy samples). This sends a clear message to sample collection staff that their process must be improved. The laboratory must have a clear procedure that is followed to handle such situations. You may have different procedures depending on whether the sample can be easily collected (e.g., surgical biopsies or CSF versus a simple blood draw) and tests for which identification is critical (e.g., tubes for cross-matching and transfusion).

For samples such as urine, CSF, and synovial fluid, the sample reception site may be the only place where critical clinical information can be ascertained. A cloudy urine or dark CSF can provide the client with clues to the patient's condition. Once samples pass through sample reception and are placed into auto-analyzers, the opportunity to harvest this information is lost.

5.4.7 Pre-examination Handling, Preparation and Storage

The laboratory shall have procedures and appropriate facilities for securing patient samples and avoiding deterioration, loss or damage during pre-examination activities and during handling, preparation and storage.

Laboratory procedures shall include time limits for requesting additional examinations or further examinations on the same primary sample.

REMARKS

Problems and accidents happen. Samples are going to be improperly stored. Trays of samples will be dropped. The one point of 5.4.7 is simple: bad things occur. In order to minimize these risks:

1. Proactively look at all your systems to minimize all types of risks
2. Make sure you have systems in place to ensure that staff and management know when a problem happens
3. React in a manner that best mitigates the damage to patient care

When a sample is damaged, lost, or destroyed, the most important issues are time and quality communications. We suggest your protocols include quick and personal contact with the client. Sending an email may be considered efficient at the time, but explaining what happened over the phone is better while face-to-face is always best.

Personal communication not only helps calm emotions but is also useful for retrieving essential information such as:

a) Is this an urgent specimen?
b) Is the patient available for re-sampling?
c) Is the delay in testing going to impact clinical decisions?

If delay in testing results in potential or actual increased morbidity and mortality, we suggest that it be your laboratory's policy to reference this in your quality meetings and consider it for inclusion in your hospital sentinel event discussions, if available. Remember, mistakes are opportunities to learn, not a time to blame (at least for the first time).

The other important aspect of 5.4.7 is that the laboratory treat samples properly for accurate testing. Are samples stored in the laboratory at the right temperature? Are specimens tested while they are within manufacturer's or lab's validated stability timeframe? Are they kept in such a way to prevent contamination? Are you storing them properly and long enough to handle a future add-on request from the clinician or for retesting if the clinician questions the original result?

Why being in compliance with this FOS is important:

The process of transporting, receiving, and preparing patient specimens include many people and multiple locations. With each step and each person, risk increases. The only reliable way to decrease this risk is through the creation and maintenance of systems, training people on how these systems work, and learning from mistakes that will inevitably happen.

If you lack adequate systems, creating and maintaining proper transport, reception and processing procedures may be the most important thing you can do to improve your laboratory's impact on productivity, patient outcomes, and staff safety.

Materials Included In This FOS
• Specimen Transportation, Reception and Handling Policies and Procedures
• Patient Reception Log
• Specimen Transport Policy
• Specimen Reception Procedure and Criteria
• Specimen Handling Log

FOS: Quality Indicators / ISO 4.14.7

4.14.7 Quality Indicators

The laboratory shall establish quality indicators to monitor and evaluate performance throughout critical aspects of pre-examination, examination and post-examination processes.

EXAMPLE: Number of unacceptable samples, number of errors at registration and/or accession, number of corrected reports.

The process of monitoring quality indicators shall be planned, which includes establishing the objectives, methodology, interpretation, limits, action plan and duration of measurement.

The indicators shall be periodically reviewed, to ensure their continued appropriateness.

NOTE 1: Quality indicators to monitor non-examination procedures, such as laboratory safety and environment, completeness of equipment and personnel records, and effectiveness of the document control system may provide valuable management insights.

NOTE 2: The laboratory should establish quality indicators for systematically monitoring and evaluating the laboratory's contribution to patient care (see 4.12).

The laboratory, in consultation with the users, shall establish turnaround times for each of its examinations that reflect clinical needs. The laboratory shall periodically evaluate whether or not it is meeting the established turnaround times.

REMARKS

It's useful to think of creating and maintaining Quality Management Systems (QMS) as a cascade of events. First, you have a Quality Policy to provide overall guidance. The next step is to provide Quality Objectives describing specific areas of desired improvement. This stage is followed by one in which you create specific, quantifiable Quality Indicators to drive your objectives forward.

Your Quality Objectives and Quality Indicators are determined by evaluating these Objectives and Indicators both in terms of fixing problems and also in terms of improvement. Lastly, you must develop target values or performance thresholds for all of your Quality Indicators. Improvement can occur in several forms such as increases in productivity, safety, economic and—most of all—elevating how the laboratory's work can improve patient outcomes.

Pre-analytical steps including sample collection are often the most important to ensuring quality testing results. No amount of laboratory QMS efforts can fix a specimen which is of poor quality at the start. While many of these pre-analytical quality indicators are outside of the laboratory's direct control, you can have an impact on improving these monitors. If your clients are not meeting thresholds for specimen labeling or acceptability, further analysis is indicated. You may need to drill down to find out if this is a problem associated to just a few clients or to many clients. Depending on the problem identified, general educational materials or training for specific clients may be necessary.

Why being in compliance with this FOS is important:

The sample collection department is the face of the laboratory, and striving to increase quality through ongoing identification and implementation of quality indicators can help improve the patient experience, decrease errors, and improve the contribution the laboratory makes towards delivering quality patient outcomes.

Areas of desired improvement and the decreasing of risks can only be actionable with a plan and actions. Not executing a quality indicator program will lead to not fixing known problems and not improving upon known areas. This will lead directly to errors and accidents. Executing an effective quality indicator program will drive specific actions that will decrease error, increase productivity, safety and patient outcomes. This is perhaps the most important aspect of your quality journey.

Materials Included In This FOS
• Quality Indicators Policies and Procedures
• Quality Indicators Worksheet

QUALITY ASSURANCE

FOS: Customer & Employee Feedback / ISO 4.8, 4.14.3, 4.14.4

4.8 Resolution of Complaints

The laboratory shall have a documented procedure for the management of complaints or other feedback received from clinicians, patients, laboratory staff or other parties. Records shall be maintained of all complaints and their investigation and the action taken (see also 4.14.3).

REMARKS

It is human nature to view complaints as something negative—not to mention a distraction from your primary work. But, taken another way, complaints are an excellent source of information and can yield important clues about how to improve the quality of your operations. View them as opportunities for improvement and ways to better meet your users' needs. Complaints also offer an important opportunity to communicate with staff, clients, other hospital departments, and the community.

When receiving a complaint, carefully listen, try to fully understand the issue, and document the encounter. For complaints where timing is important (such as an alleged error impacting patient care), you need to respond as quickly as you do thoroughly. Ensure that you have a way to feed this information into your process for nonconformities, including the potential need to halt testing.

Regardless of the kind of complaint, there are a few universal things you need to do. First and foremost, write everything down. There are many ways of reporting complaints, but typically complaint logs will contain the following minimum criteria:

1) Description of the complaint
2) Investigation records
3) Resolution

There are sample templates available for both client-generated and staff-generated complaints.

4.14.3 Assessment of User Feedback

The laboratory shall seek information relating to user perception as to whether the service has met the needs and requirements of users. The methods for obtaining and using this information shall include cooperation with users or their representatives in monitoring the laboratory's performance, provided that the laboratory ensures confidentiality to other users. Records shall be kept of information collected and actions taken.

REMARKS

User feedback can take many forms and range from complaints to casual comments from clients. Your staff needs to be instructed to listen for positive and negative feedback and report anything they feel is important. Feedback can also be collected from staff and client satisfaction surveys. Regardless of the source, feedback should be recorded, all stakeholders should be able to access it, and the contents should be assessed on whether corrective action is required and whether it should be included as a quality objective or indicator.

4.14.4 Staff Suggestions

Laboratory management shall encourage staff to make suggestions for the improvement of any aspect of the laboratory service. Suggestions shall be evaluated, implemented as appropriate and feedback provided to the staff. Records of suggestions and actions taken by the management shall be maintained.

REMARKS

Your staff should be encouraged to voice complaints. The reality, however, is that staff typically fear complaining due to fear of retribution from superiors or other staff. When staff wish to come forward with a complaint or suggestion, it needs to be handled with sensitivity. It is recommended that your lab have an open policy regarding complaints and suggestions. Staff must believe such feedback is welcome; a well-defined procedure that ensures confidentiality is a major aspect of that.

Having a suggestion box in the lab can also be an excellent way for staff to anonymously put forward complaints or suggestions. However, you must evaluate the effectiveness of your suggestion methods. An empty suggestion box does not mean there are no issues; instead, it means that you must do more to solicit staff suggestions.

This is not to say that every employee suggestion must be implemented. The laboratory management should have a process to evaluate each suggestion. Feedback on the suggestions is mandatory. This is especially important if the suggestion is not implemented. The rationale must be explained to the staff, or the management may be accused of not listening, and this will depress morale and decrease future suggestions.

It is ideal that all complaints be addressed at quality meetings and, assuming it is not a confidential or staff-related issue, shared among the staff as a first-rate learning opportunity.

Complaints are also an excellent way to identify items for new quality objectives and indicators.

Lastly, the results of staff suggestions must be communicated to at least the person who voiced the suggestion, if not the entire laboratory.

Why being in compliance with this FOS is important:

Being open to suggestions, listening, and understanding are the first steps to improvement. Complaints and suggestions from staff and clients as well as staff and client satisfaction surveys are perhaps your best resource to gather ideas for quality indicators and improvement.

Failing to do this will hurt your reputation and effectiveness. A defensive attitude can do a great deal of harm. Doing it well will help your laboratory recognize and resolve safety issues, help create a productive work environment, and even positively impact the quality of patient care.

Materials Included In This FOS
• Customer and Employee Feedback Policies and Procedures
• Complaint Log
• Client Satisfaction Survey
• Staff Satisfaction Survey

FOS: Adverse Incident Reporting / ISO 5.3.2.6, 5.3.1.6

5.3.2.6 Reagents and Consumables – Adverse Incident Reporting

Adverse incidents and accidents that can be attributed directly to specific reagents or consumables shall be investigated and reported to the manufacturer and appropriate authorities, as required.

REMARKS

There are two issues here. One is maintaining compliance with local laws. The other is your ethical responsibility to report reagent or system problems so that manufacturers know a problem exists and can take appropriate action. Most manufacturers take quality problems very seriously, but they cannot possibly understand every single variable. Whether you like it or not, YOU, the laboratory client, act as the ultimate quality control for the manufacturer. Manufacturers and labs must act as good partners because your goals are the same: providing the highest level of patient care possible.

Because Adverse Incidents are typically identified at the department level, 5.3.2.6 and 5.3.1.6 are listed in the Technical Departments as well. Having said that, the quality department must take the lead in creating, enforcing, and documenting rules and guidelines for adverse incident reporting. We encourage you to work closely with department managers. If you feel a particular department manager is not up to the task, it needs to be communicated to the laboratory director. He should consider if the quality department should take primary responsibility.

5.3.1.6 Equipment Adverse Incidence Reporting

Adverse incidents and accidents that can be attributed directly to specific equipment shall be investigated and reported to the manufacturer and appropriate authorities, as required.

REMARKS

If a problem with an instrument and/or reagent system occurs, it is almost certain the same problem has or will occur at other labs, too. It should be a part of all our missions to help manufacturers identify problems so they can rectify them and—most importantly—notify other labs before the problem affects more patients. If you want to have a positive impact on the global patient population, identifying problems quickly and immediately reporting them to the manufacturer is a great start. It is possible you could save lives. In most jurisdictions, manufacturers are required to report adverse events resulting from any use of their systems potentially impacting patient care. Depending on the kind and scope of the problem, the offending product may be recalled or caution notifications issued to all client labs around the world. As a consumer of lab products, you are a partner in ensuring the safety and efficacy of laboratory products worldwide.

In some regions, you are required to report certain defects directly to regulatory authorities. If you believe a problem is serious enough, and/or you do not believe the manufacturer is taking your complaints seriously enough, it may be your responsibility to report to the local government for possible action.

Because Adverse Incidents are typically identified at the department level, 5.3.2.6 and 5.3.1.6 are listed in the Technical Departments as well. Having said that, the quality department must take the lead in creating, enforcing, and documenting rules and guidelines for adverse incident reporting. We encourage you to work closely with department managers. If you feel a particular department manager is not up to the task, it needs to be communicated to the laboratory director. He should consider if the quality department should take primary responsibility.

Sometimes, these incidents result from a combination of specific reagents on a specific instrument. If these are obtained from different manufacturers, both must be notified.

Lastly, if you receive a recall notice from the manufacturer, you must have a process in place to handle such an occurrence. This may involve temporary cessation of testing, modification of procedures or reagents, investigation of effect on already released results, and the recall of results. As always, you must follow the manufacturer's instructions.

Why being in compliance with this FOS is important:

Identifying, investigating, and reporting problems will not only impact your laboratory and patient populations but, when combined with the manufacturer or regulatory authority, may impact the healthcare industry across the globe.

Materials Included In This FOS
• Adverse Incident Reporting Policies and Procedures
• Adverse Incident Reporting Letter to Manufacturer
• Recall Policies and Procedures

FOS: Inter-Laboratory Comparisons / ISO 5.6.3, 5.6.3.1, 5.6.3.2, 5.6.3.3, 5.6.3.4

5.6.3 Inter-Laboratory Comparisons

5.6.3.1 Participation

The laboratory shall participate in an inter-laboratory comparison program(s) such as external quality assessment program or proficiency testing program appropriate to the examination and interpretations of examination results. The laboratory shall monitor the results of the inter-laboratory comparison program(s) and participate in the implementation of corrective actions when predetermined performance criteria are not fulfilled.

NOTE: The laboratory should participate in inter-laboratory comparison programs that substantially fulfill the relevant requirements of ISO/IEC 17043.

The laboratory shall establish a documented procedure for inter-laboratory comparison participation that includes defined responsibilities and instructions for participation, and any performance criteria that differ from the criteria used in the inter-laboratory comparison program.

Inter-laboratory comparison program(s) chosen by the laboratory shall, as far as possible, provide clinically relevant challenges that mimic patient samples and have the effect of checking the entire examination process, including pre-examination procedures and post-examination procedures, where possible.

REMARKS

Inter-laboratory comparison programs are also referred to as proficiency testing (PT) programs.

Many professionals consider rigorous PT programs to be one of the most important parts of operating a quality laboratory. Why? Because PT programs represent the chance for one lab to blindly compare all of its internal variables against statistically relevant peer groupings on a per-test methodology basis. To underline the importance of PT, manufacturers and regulatory authorities consistently scour published external PT data to identify possible lapses in their quality systems.

The over 7,000 global College of American Pathologists (CAP)-accredited laboratories, for example, are required to run PT on all tests several times a year. Failure to successfully participate may lead to suspension of a lab's accreditation or requirements to cease some areas of laboratory testing. If CAP PT programs are available in your area, you have no excuse not to participate in external PT for all your tests. Although utilizing CAP PT is not an ISO 15189 requirement, we believe it is one of the best investments you can make.

The best way to negate value from a PT program (and to jeopardize your laboratory's accreditation) is to treat a PT specimen in a manner differently from patient samples (e.g., run it several times, only let certain lab employees perform the testing, and/or perhaps compare results with a manufacturer's rep or friendly lab). Not only would doing this defeat the purpose of using PT, it may mean failing to identify some systemic problem in a manufactured assay system itself.

In some major jurisdictions, cheating on a PT is a crime (fraud). In addition to sanction on the laboratory, loss of accreditation or closure, the individuals and director may also be punished (by the loss of professional licensure, a fine, or even jail).

Most regulatory agencies also have a strict prohibition on communication about PT data or the sharing of PT samples. Ensure your laboratory has a prohibition on such communication until after the deadline for submission of results and that your laboratory notifies appropriate authorities if they ever receive PT samples from another laboratory.

Many manufacturers have inter-laboratory comparison programs available for their customers. These may be appropriate but may also have limitations. These limitations include the fact that, in many cases, samples consist of excess control and calibrator materials that are not representative of normal biological samples. Also, the manufacturers of PT program materials tend to use unnaturally optimized materials that again may not be representative of typical biological specimens and do not challenge potential matrix effects. Some also claim a potential conflict of interest by making them too easy to pass and thus makes manufacturers of PT programs suspect.

Some for-profit manufacturers sell external PT materials. These can be excellent, but purchasers must ensure they don't get a matrix effect from preservatives or other artificial materials. (Some manufacturers use preservatives to promote a longer shelf life and increased commercial viability.)

We recommend not-for-profit commercial PT suppliers. The world's largest—and arguably the most rigorous—program is administered by CAP. CAP has PT materials for over 1,000 different tests. They also have highly sophisticated analytic procedures that segment results into peer groupings. Over 23,000 clinical laboratories in 72 countries utilize CAP PT programs, and we recommend searching for CAP PT programs available in your area*.
For purposes of transparency, the producer of LEAP software is also the representative of CAP PT programs in Japan.

5.6.3.2 Alternative Approaches

Whenever an inter-laboratory comparison is not available, the laboratory shall develop other approaches and provide objective evidence for determining the acceptability of examination results.

Whenever possible, this mechanism shall utilize appropriate materials.

NOTE: Examples of such materials include:
- Certified reference materials;
- Samples previously examined;
- Materials from cell or tissue repositories;
- Exchange of samples with other laboratories;
- Control materials that are tested daily in inter-laboratory comparison programs.

REMARKS

Note that 5.3.2.6 is only applicable if external inter-laboratory comparison programs are *not* available.

There are times when alternative programs are appropriate and necessary, such as when you are using a laboratory-developed assay and externally administered programs are unavailable. Another example would be an assay system that is rare or very new and for which no external programs have been developed. Some distributive test models (such as using bioinformatics analysis at a second lab) are not able to use commercial PT programs because of the prohibition on intra-laboratory comparison. And, if you are one of those unlucky laboratories who still perform bleeding time (and, these days, why are you still doing this test?), it is not a test that allows for external PT. Lastly, some interpretive tests, such as surgical specimens or cytology, are dependent on the competency of those individuals who perform the interpretation. In such instances, a quality peer review program is required to ensure accurate results are reported.

5.6.3.3 Analysis of Inter-Laboratory Comparison Samples

The laboratory shall integrate inter-laboratory comparison samples into the routine workflow in a manner that follows, as much as possible, the handling of patient samples.

Inter-laboratory comparison samples shall be examined by personnel who routinely examine patient samples using the same procedures as those used for samples.

The laboratory shall not communicate with other participants in the inter-laboratory comparison program about sample data until after the date for submission of data.

The laboratory shall not refer inter-laboratory comparison samples for confirmatory examination before submission of the data, although this would routinely be done with patient samples.

5.6.3.4 Evaluation of Laboratory Performance

The performance in inter-laboratory comparisons shall be reviewed and discussed with relevant staff.

When predetermined performance criteria are not fulfilled (i.e., nonconformities are present), staff shall participate in the implementation and recording of corrective action. The effectiveness of corrective action shall be monitored. The returned results shall be evaluated for trends that indicate potential nonconformities and preventative action shall be taken.

REMARKS

The main point here is to underline that *the only time you can be absolutely sure your tests are accurate is at the point of* ***inter-laboratory comparison***. Also, intervals of time between inter-laboratory comparisons need to be considered suspect because they are only being judged by internally regulated systems. This is especially true when any changes of any time occur—and the bigger the change, the bigger the risk. Changes can include relatively routine things like new lots of reagents, calibrators, and control as well as major changes like a new assay coming into service or instrument replacements. To reiterate: the only time you can be absolutely confident of your results is after you participate and complete in an inter-laboratory comparison program.

If your laboratory has a history of no discrepancies on your inter-laboratory comparison program(s), you need to investigate why? *All* quality laboratories have discrepancies in inter-laboratory comparison results. When discrepancies are identified, this is a real opportunity for improvement.

The first thing you need to do when investigating PT discrepancies is to review for clerical errors. You should examine the Discrepancy Report and all documentation and worksheets (paper and electronic). Evaluate if all the units were reported correctly, if the decimal point was entered into the correct place, were there accurate records of which peer group should be used for comparison, and whether there was a transcription error. A great many PT discrepancies are actually reporting errors.

If the paperwork is problem free, the next thing to do is to check available data on or about the time the PT sample was tested. What was the calibration status? Were patient results trending high or low? How about QC trends or major instrument maintenance/repairs? Who was doing the testing that day? As you move forward in your investigation, every puzzle piece counts.

We always recommend you save excess PT materials. Preferably, store them in the freezer to keep them as stable as possible, and also so you can retest them to compare results with those already reported. This alone could solve the mystery. Remember, however, that many PT samples are shipped without preservatives because they are designed to mimic normal patient samples as closely as possible and avoid, for example, the matrix effect. For this and other reasons, all PT samples stored for long periods of time prior to re-testing should be considered suspect.

The laboratory's performance for any PT challenge that was intended to be graded, but was not for any reason, needs to be evaluated by the laboratory. No matter what the cause for the inability to be graded (e.g., lack of consensus, delay in returning the laboratory's analysis), the laboratory must determine if its performance is acceptable or not. If not acceptable, the laboratory must perform a root-cause analysis just as it would for a graded, missed challenge.

If your investigation finds a systemic problem, you may need to review your patient results to see if any were affected. This should be done in conjunction with the medical director. If reported results were invalid, you will need to recall those results.

After you investigate a discrepant PT result, you will need to report your findings and detail the problem, including all investigation steps taken. If you discovered nothing, you will need to report this as an outlier or random error and henceforth pay special attention to the future performance of this assay. Note that this conclusion can only be reached when you exclude all other potential causes.

Multiple sequential PT failures may be the result of a systemic failure in your laboratory, and the situation needs to be disclosed, discussed, and forward action determined at the highest level. This forward action may include ceasing testing and sending the assay to a referral laboratory until the problem is resolved.

Why being in compliance with this FOS is important:

Internal quality control is done within the isolation of your own laboratory systems. If there are fundamental problems in these internal systems, and you do not check this with external comparisons, it is possible you are reporting suboptimal results forever. We have, in fact, seen this occur where a laboratory reported out more than 200,000 results over a decade with a 20% negative bias. They (and especially the new quality manager) were pretty shocked when they did their first inter-laboratory comparison.

Materials Included In This FOS
• Inter-Laboratory Comparisons Policies and Procedures
• Inter-Laboratory Comparison Program Plan
• Inter-Laboratory Comparisons Evaluation

FOS: Evaluation & Audits / ISO 4.14, 4.14.1, 4.14.5, 4.14.8

4.14 Evaluation and Audits

4.14.1 General

The laboratory shall plan and implement the evaluation and internal audit processes needed to:

a) Demonstrate the pre-examination, examination, and post-examination and supporting processes are being conducted in a manner that meets the needs and requirements of users;
b) Ensure conformity to the quality management system;
c) Continually improve the effectiveness of the quality management system;
d) The results of evaluation and improvement activities shall be included in the input to the management review (see 4.15).

NOTE: For improvement activities, see 4.10, 4.11 and 4.12.

4.14.5 Internal Audit

The laboratory shall conduct internal audits at planned intervals to determine whether all activities in the quality management system, including pre-examination, examination, and post-examination:

a) Conform to requirements of this International Standard and to requirements established by the laboratory, and
b) Are implemented, effective, and maintained.

NOTE 1: The cycle for internal auditing should normally be completed in one year. It is not necessary that internal audits cover each year, in depth, all elements of the quality management system. The laboratory may decide to focus on a particular activity without completely neglecting the others.

Audits shall be conducted by personnel trained to assess the performance of managerial and technical processes of the quality management system.

The audit program shall take into account the status and importance of the processes and technical and management areas to be audited, as well as the results of previous audits. The audit criteria, scope, frequency, and methods shall be defined and documented.

NOTE 2: See ISO 19011 for guidance

The laboratory shall have a documented procedure to define the responsibilities and requirements for planning and conducting audits, and for reporting results and maintaining records (see 4.13).

Personnel responsible for the area being audited shall ensure that appropriate action is promptly undertaken when nonconformities are identified. Corrective action shall be taken without undue delay to eliminate the causes of the detected nonconformities (see 4.10).

REMARKS

If you lack special training, we highly recommend working with a trained professional or organization to set up and run your internal auditing processes. This will typically include creating a checklist. We also recommend that you work with someone experienced for your first few internal audits. An effective internal audit is not just about "ticking boxes". Rather, it is about understanding how your underlying systems are functioning day to day.

There are different philosophies about scheduled versus unscheduled audits. Although it is your decision as to how to proceed, as a general rule the first few audits probably should be scheduled. A schedule gives your staff time to review and address systems prior to the internal audit—which can be very positive in the early days of your QMS journey. In time, however, you may want to consider unscheduled internal audits because in order to obtain real value from your QMS you will need to remain in continuous compliance, 24/7. If your lab is in compliance only in preparation and during an internal or external audit period, you accrue all the cost and work of creating and managing a QMS program with few of the benefits. An audit should reflect your actual day-to-day process and not an artificial state.

LEAP is designed to help you gain and maintain continuous compliance in your QMS 24/7. If you use LEAP as directed, you will be able to detect a breach in your system as soon as it occurs since the QMS Dashboard will notify you when you are out of compliance. LEAP will allow you to identify the department in which the discrepancy occurred, what the discrepancy is (through the department-specific QMS Dashboard), and where corrective measures should be instituted.

Just like complaints or reporting nonconformities, audit findings help the lab to improve processes, procedures, and quality. An audit that repeatedly finds no gap may make the department feel good, but it is largely a waste of effort and has not improved your laboratory's quality.

For bad audits, an immediate search for a scapegoat is likewise not very useful. It is more often than not a process or system issue rather than the fault of an individual. It is best to work together to find a solution.

Lastly, auditors must be trained to perform audits, and objectivity and impartiality must be part of the audit process. Audits also should be independent of the area being audited. This is best done by someone from an independent quality team or someone working in a department different from the one being audited.

4.14.8 Reviews by External Organizations

When reviews by external organizations indicate the laboratory has nonconformities or potential nonconformities, the laboratory shall take appropriate immediate actions and, as warranted, corrective action or preventative action to ensure continuing compliance with the requirements of this International Standard. Records shall be kept of the reviews and of the corrective actions and preventative actions taken.

NOTE: Examples of reviews by external accreditation organizations include: onsite user evaluations, accreditation assessments, regulatory agencies' inspections, and health and safety inspections.

REMARKS

Please refer to the remarks on 4.14.5 about internal audits as all these comments apply equally to external audits.

External audits should be seen as an opportunity for fresh eyes to review your QMS processes. This way, you can confirm your system is working, as well as gain new perspectives and insights. Remember, your auditors visit many labs and see a wide variety of methods—both good and bad—so their knowledge base is broad. Finally, don't forget to ask probing questions and try to get as much as possible out of the investment you are making in the audit process.

It is also helpful if your staff can perform audits of external laboratories. This can be done by participating in accrediting agency peer audits or through informal agreements within or between laboratories. This can be a valuable way to bring some new ideas and processes to your own laboratory. Try to take advantage of all such opportunities.

A fully functioning LEAP can also greatly help you maximize the effectiveness of your external audit. If you correctly populate each of your evidence folders, most of the documented evidence will be available for examination by your external auditor within LEAP. You may also want to consider giving the external auditor access to LEAP during—and perhaps even prior to—the audit. This will give them the opportunity to review all your documentation (if they understand the same language), maximizing the time they spend interacting with your staff. We stress again that an external audit gives you and your staff a prime chance to work with and learn from experts of vast experience and knowledge. Note that you can activate an "inspector" role in LEAP for this purpose. The inspector will have access to all the information stored within LEAP, but they will not have the permission to change any content.

It is only human nature to seek a "good score" on an external audit or any kind of test. However, a perfect result has little value and probably represents a superficial review. Each opportunity for improvement should be seen as helpful. Remember, unless there is an immediate threat to patient or staff safety, you will be given the opportunity to take corrective actions by an external auditor. Do not, however, use this as a license to be unprepared for an external audit—experienced auditors can smell an unprepared lab a mile away. Also, an auditor has limited time and, if overwhelmed by large numbers of easily correctable deficiencies, they may not have time to find all the things that can truly help your laboratory. It is best never to leave anything to chance.

Why being in compliance with this FOS is important:

The internal audit acts as a barometer as to how your laboratory's QMS system is performing. It also allows for open communication, helping to identify points requiring improvement. The external auditing process does the same thing, but from a different, "external" perspective. Internal and external audits act as one of the cornerstones of your QMS, giving you a constant influx of information and supplying your staff meaningful targets for improvement.

Materials Included In This FOS
• Evaluation and Audits Policies and Procedures
• Internal Audit Checklist

FOS: External Services & Supplies / ISO 4.6

4.6 External Services and Supplies

The laboratory shall have a documented procedure for the selection and purchasing of external services, equipment, reagents and consumable supplies that affect the quality of its services (see also 5.3).

The laboratory shall select and approve suppliers based on their ability to supply external services, equipment, reagents and consumable supplies in accordance with the laboratory's requirements; however, it may be necessary to collaborate with other organizational departments or functions to fulfill this requirement. Criteria for selection shall be established.

A list of selected and approved suppliers of equipment, reagents and consumables shall be maintained.

Purchasing information shall describe the requirements for the product or service to be purchased.

The laboratory shall monitor the performance of suppliers to ensure that purchased services or items consistently meet the stated criteria.

REMARKS

This section is essentially asking if you have considered and documented a process whereby you can determine which vendors to buy from and why. To satisfy the terms of this FOS, you need to document your system for choosing vendors and read through the ISO 15189 requirements listed below and add them to your Vendor Management Protocol.

You should also decide what to include in your Vendor Contractual Agreements. Often, vendors will have their own contracts they want you to sign, but please remember that such vendor-generated contracts usually exist to serve their best interests and not yours. As such, you should consider your objectives in entering into such an agreement. Do you want to be able to exit the agreement in case of poor vendor performance? And what about price guarantees? If contracts include a service component, you may want to ensure there are provisions protecting the confidentiality of patient data. You may also require service representatives to submit detailed reports on services rendered. As you can see, the scope of such agreements is wide. The use of legal advice or counsel is strongly encouraged to assist in the drafting and reviewing of contracts, especially for a new lab and initial set up.

Sample Vendor Management Protocols are included within this FOS. Of course, these may or may not be appropriate for your laboratory, and you should note that these serve only as samples.

Lastly, it is understandable that many of your vendor relationships may be long-term and personal. Now that you have begun your QMS journey, this is an excellent opportunity to create a checklist and explain to all your vendors the ISO 15189 requirements that you are going to have to comply with and thereby vet their services to ensure the best use of funds for the betterment of patients. You should also point out that this vetting process will need to be repeated on a regular basis. In some cases, this process may even help your laboratory earn better business conditions and even improve your personal relationships.

Why being in compliance with this FOS is important:

Failing to manage processes for purchasing external services and supplies can lead to wasteful purchases, can be an opportunity for employees to profit or receive favors from vendors while costing the laboratory money, and/or not receive the proper services and supplies. These potentially non-optimal products and services can lead to errors and loss of productivity. Nothing is more frustrating than having to cease patient testing and communicating such service interruptions to your users due to lack of supplies.

Materials Included In This FOS
• External Services and Supplies Policies and Procedures
• Vendor Checklist
• Vendor Service Agreement Template
• Approved Vendor List

FOS: Advisory Services / ISO 4.7

4.7 Advisory Services

The laboratory shall establish arrangements for communicating with users on the following:

a) Advising on choice of examinations and use of the services, including required type of sample (see also 5.4), clinical indications and limitations of examination procedures and the frequency of requesting the examination;
b) Advising on individual clinical cases;
c) Professional judgements on the interpretation of the results of examination (see 5.1.2 and 5.1.6);
d) Promoting the effective utilization of laboratory services;
e) Consulting on scientific and logistic matters such as instances of failure of sample(s) to meet acceptable criteria.

REMARKS

Part of your advisory services can be enshrined in your testing handbook, on your website, and through written instructions to your laboratory. There are two other kinds of advisory services you need to consider. The first is general test information for when your laboratory adopts a new methodology or brings on a new assay. In such cases, advisory services are a form of education to help clients and auxiliary staff understand the limitations of an assay, its sample requirements, and how to interpret the data. In terms of implementation, you could offer an educational program on your website or send a memo to your clients. If you want to be more proactive, however, you can provide e-learning programs complete with testing and have clients initial that they have received and understood the materials. It is always recommended that qualified people are available to field client questions and that all of these interactions are recorded.

Other advisory services concern specific cases and usually involve your medical director or qualified clinical consultant with documented, delegated authority. Since there are obviously very important interactions, they will need to be accurately recorded. Note that these represent excellent opportunities for your staff to learn new and interesting things and can be a time for an off-site medical director to interact with the laboratory.

As a clinical lab, you are part of the broader healthcare delivery team. As such, it is recommended that you look at your mission (i.e., mission statement) and determine what you can reasonably do to help improve quality patient outcomes and contribute to the economic health of the healthcare system. It must be understood, of course, that there are legal and even cultural issues involved, but the goal should be for your laboratory to do more than just generate data, and you should offer added value. When discussing advisory services, these are the sort of issues that need addressing.

Although we have provided a Sample Laboratory Advisory Services Template for you to review, please understand that each situation is unique, and the template should be modified accordingly. Do you have an Advisory Service Management Protocol? Is it the best it can be? How can you make it better? Is this documented? Are the advisory services provided by your medical director or delegated to a clinical consultant? Is this delegation documented?

You should carefully review the ISO 15189 standards to determine whether you are in compliance with the above questions. Outside of a pure research or epidemiological setting, we cannot envision any circumstances where a clinical laboratory would mark this FOS as N/A.

Why being in compliance with this FOS is important:

Providing quality advisory services is the difference between your laboratory merely being a generator of data or being a generator of value. You need to make clear in all your documentation to users that these services are available. Information about when and how to access these services must also be communicated to your users. And, when requests do come into the laboratory, these need to take priority over everything else. This is the time for the laboratory to shine!

Materials Included In This FOS
• Advisory Services Policies and Procedures
• List of Personnel Authorized to Provide Advisory Services
• Advisory Services Log

FOS: Sample Storage, Retention & Disposal / ISO 5.7.2

5.7.2 Storage, Retention and Disposal of Clinical Samples

The laboratory shall have documented procedure for identification, collection, retention, indexing, access, storage, maintenance and safe disposal of clinical samples.

The laboratory shall define the length of time clinical samples are to be retained. Retention time shall be defined by the nature of the sample, the examination and any applicable requirements.

NOTE: Legal liability concerns regarding certain types of procedures (e.g., histology examination, genetic examination, pediatric examination) may require the retention of certain samples for much longer periods than for other samples.

Safe disposal of samples shall be carried out in accordance with local regulations or recommendations for waste management.

REMARKS

The primary objective of 5.7.2 is to enable the laboratory to reliably re-test specimens when required. Re-testing may be required because of problems detected during QC, by physician request, or even because you are legally compelled to do so. In addition to repeating the test, you may need to perform different tests if required by your reflex test procedures or by physician request. The requirements for re-testing are as follows: you must be able to find the specimen; you must be able to confirm the identity of specimen; you must know that the specimen was stored in conditions suitable to ensure accuracy for the re-testing process; and you must ensure the re-testing occurs within your validated specimen stability window.

Note that, for larger labs, sample storage, retention, and disposal may be best managed by the use of tracking software and barcode systems. Typically, storage and collection systems are managed in conjunction with specimen collection and accession.

Why being in compliance with this FOS is important:

If a sample is disposed of prematurely and the acceptance criteria is not met and the user later requests a re-examination, the patient will need to be re-collected, which may not be possible and may result in customer dissatisfaction. This can lead to delay or a misdiagnosis and reduction in the quality of patient care. Storing samples in unsuitable environmental conditions may lead to incorrect examination results. In some cases, improperly discarding samples may expose laboratory staff, hospital staff, and/or the community to dangerous pathogens or chemicals. There may be legal requirements related to the disposal of some specimens that can relate to the ethical treatment of human samples (see 4.1.1.3 (d)). Lastly, specimens may be labeled with confidential or protected patient information that may require specific disposal procedures (see 4.1.1.3 (e)).

Materials Included In This FOS
• Sample Storage, Retention and Disposal Policies and Procedures
• Criteria for Sample Storage, Retention, and Disposal
• Sample Log Sheet

FOS: Service Agreements / ISO 4.4, 4.4.1, 4.4.2

4.4 Service Agreements

4.4.1 Establishment of Service Agreements

The laboratory shall have documented procedures for the establishment and review of agreements for providing medical laboratory services.

Each request accepted by the laboratory for examination(s) shall be considered an agreement.

Agreements to provide medical laboratory services shall take into account the request, the examination and the report. The agreement shall specify the information needed on the request to ensure appropriate examination and result interpretation.

The following conditions shall be met when the laboratory enters into an agreement to provide medical laboratory services:

a) The requirements of the customers and users, and of the provider of the laboratory service, including the examination processes to be used, shall be defined, documented and understood (see 5.4.2 and 5.5);
b) The laboratory shall have the capability and resources to meet the requirements;
c) Laboratory personnel shall have the skills and expertise necessary for the performance of the intended examinations;
d) Examination procedures selected shall be appropriate and able to meet the customers' needs (see 5.5.1);
e) Customers and users shall be informed of deviations from the agreement that impact upon the examination results;
f) Reference shall be made to any work referred by the laboratory to a referral laboratory or consultant.

NOTE 1: Customers and users may include clinicians, healthcare organizations, third party payment organizations or agencies, pharmaceutical companies, and patients.

NOTE 2: Where patients are customers (e.g., when patients have the ability to directly request examinations), changes in service should be reflected in explanatory information and laboratory reports.

NOTE 3: Laboratories should not enter into financial arrangements with referring practitioners or funding agencies where those arrangements act as an inducement for the referral of examinations or patients or interfere with the practitioner's independent assessment of what is best for the patient.

REMARKS

The objective is clear communication between the lab and its users about mutual responsibilities and expectations. If your lab is hospital-based and the samples you test are limited to those generated at your hospital, these service agreement requirements are generally managed within your Laboratory Test Guide and reporting forms. If you accept reference samples, you will also want to consider an additional written agreement between the laboratory and the user, and not just the Laboratory Test Guide and reporting forms. This agreement can cover areas such as defining limitations of liability, financial terms and conditions, and general contractual terms and conditions.

As a reminder, every completed requisition form (paper or electronic) represents an agreement for the laboratory to provide services to the user. As such, they are all service agreements. These requisition forms must clearly indicate which testing is to be performed by the laboratory and which will be sent to a referral laboratory.

4.4.2 Review of Service Agreements

Reviews of agreements to provide medical laboratory services shall include all aspects of the agreement. Records of these reviews shall include any changes to the agreement and any pertinent discussions.

When an agreement needs to be amended after laboratory services have commenced, the same agreement review process shall be repeated and any amendments shall be communicated to all affected parties.

REMARKS

This usually refers to reviewing your Laboratory Test Guide, requisition forms, reporting forms, and any external agreements on a regular basis (typically once a year) or in cases where there are significant changes requiring immediate attention. All of these reviews are covered in other areas within ISO standards and LEAP. The key is to make sure the changes are universal. That is, for example, you add an assay to your available menu (or make changes to methodologies that may affect results), this needs to be addressed in the Laboratory Test Guide, on the requisition form, on the reporting form, and any possible changes to business terms (such as pricing) in case you are acting as a referral laboratory.

Why being in compliance with this FOS is important:

The creation and review of service agreements, at its most basic level, is simply clear communication between the lab and users. This increases laboratory transparency, defines expectations of both users and the laboratory, and clarifies responsibilities. The benefit is a high quality, productive relationship that helps maximize productivity, improves customer satisfaction, improves quality, and minimizes the possibility of waste and medical errors.

Materials Included In This FOS
• Service Agreements Policies and Procedures
• Laboratory Services Agreement Template

FOS: Reviewing & Reporting Results / ISO 5.7, 5.7.1, 5.8, 5.8.1, 5.8.2, 5.8.3, 5.9, 5.9.1, 5.9.2, 5.9.3

5.7 Post-Examination Processes

5.7.1 Review of Results

The laboratory shall have procedures to ensure that authorized personnel review the results of examinations before release and evaluate them against internal quality control and, as appropriate, available clinical information and previous examination results.

When the procedures for reviewing results involves automatic selection and reporting, review criteria shall be established, approved and documented (see 5.9.1).

REMARKS

Unless you are using auto-verification systems, checking the results of your quality control (QC) data prior to reporting results is intuitive enough. As a QMS-managed laboratory, you must ensure this QC review is documented with: a) the time the review was made, and b) who confirmed the results. The laboratory QMS should determine the qualifications of those allowed to review and confirm QC. For example, certain procedures may require a certified medical technologist. The authority to perform this review must be delegated in writing.

Acquiring and recording available clinical information begins with your ability to gain permission from clients to input all requested data fields. For inpatients, this data may already be available on your LIS (laboratory information systems) or HIS (hospital information systems). If you are depending on your clients to provide this data, we recommend educating them on its importance (by contacting them to supply needed information or possibly rejecting samples that lack the minimum required patient information). The more complete the clinical information you have about a patient, the more valuable your potential contribution can be. For example, if you know a patient is on immunosuppressants, a slight elevation in WBC may trigger a panic value and/or trigger you to confirm the results with a blood smear and microscopy. Clinical data can affect the results and not just the reference range (GFR calculations, MSAFP calculations, etc.).

Using results from past tests is one area in which you can be very self-reliant. Also, by contrasting recent results with those from past examinations (delta checking), you can ascertain and improve quality. One way of using past results prior to reporting is to identify erroneous results. For example, let us assume a patient has several test results for quantitate B-HCG and your results indicate a decrease in B-HCG levels. During this process, you may note that the patient is in her third trimester; therefore, it may be wise to consider re-examining the specimen prior to reporting as it may have been mislabeled or somehow switched the results. If your initial results were incorrect, you just saved the doctor and patient days of anguish. If you are right, you have confirmed something important. Of course, the only way to be certain is to review prior results (assuming appropriate clinical information is provided, of course). Please note that there are software systems that do this assessment automatically. Delta checks are also often used with auto-verification systems.

5.8 Reporting Results

5.8.1 General

The results of each examination shall be reported accurately, clearly, unambiguously and in accordance with any specific instructions in the examination procedures.

The laboratory shall define the format and medium of the report (i.e., electronic or paper) and the manner in which it is to be communicated from the laboratory.

The laboratory shall have a procedure to ensure the correctness of transcription of laboratory results.

Reports shall include the information necessary for the interpretation of the examination results.

The laboratory shall have a process notifying the requester when an examination is delayed that could compromise patient care.

5.8.2 Reporting Attributes

The laboratory shall ensure that the following report attributes effectively communicate laboratory results and meet the users' needs:

a) Comments on sample quality that might compromise examination results;
b) Comments regarding sample suitability with respect to acceptance/rejection criteria;
c) Critical results, where applicable;
d) Interpretive comments on results, where applicable, which may include the verification of the interpretation of automatically selected and reported results (see 5.9.1) in the final report.

5.8.2 Report Content

The report shall include, but not be limited to, the following:

a) A clear, unambiguous identification of the examination including, where applicable, the examination procedure;
b) The identification of the laboratory that issued the report;
c) Identification of all examinations that have been performed by a referral laboratory;
d) Patient identification and patient location on each page;
e) Name or other unique identifier of the requester and the requester's contact details;
f) Date of primary sample collection (and time, when available and relevant to patient care);
g) Type of primary sample;
h) Measurement procedure, where appropriate;
i) Examination results reported in SI units, units traceable to SI units, or other applicable units;
j) Biological reference intervals, clinical decision values, or diagrams/nomograms supporting clinical decision values, where applicable.

NOTE: Under some circumstances, it might be appropriate to distribute lists of tables of biological reference intervals to all users of laboratory services at sites where reports are received.

k) Interpretation of results, where appropriate;

   NOTE: Complete interpretation of results requires the context of clinical information that may not be available to the laboratory.

l) Other comments such as cautionary or explanatory notes (e.g., quality or adequacy of the primary sample which may have compromised results, results/interpretation from referral laboratories, use of development procedure);
m) Identification of examinations undertaken as part of a research or development program and for which no specific claims on measurement performance are available;
n) Identification of the person(s) reviewing the results and authorizing the release of the report (if not contained in the report, readily available when needed);
o) Date of the report, and time of release (if not contained in the report, readily available when needed);
p) Page number to total number of pages (e.g., "Page 1 of 5", "Page 2 of 5", etc.).

REMARKS

Complying with 5.8 means scrutinizing your patient report formats. Are the results clearly tied to the procedure name? Is the normal range aligned clearly with the results? Are abnormal results clearly identified? Is there a clear and easy way for clients to reference their results to observations or interpretive advice provided by the laboratory? Are they being transmitted accurately to an EMR or other downstream reporting system?

If your laboratory has manually transcribed something at any stage of a testing and reporting process, this means there is a high risk of transcription error. Studies have shown that even a single numeric data transcription increases the chance of a mistake from 8% to 13%. Even when double-checked, in no study does human transcription error rates approach 0%. What's more, even machine transcription is not foolproof. In fact, when machines fail, they often do so in major ways: errors in units of measurement, errors in decimal placement, and/or errors in calculated formulas repeated many times before being detected.

Imagine these kinds of errors taking place in labs all over the world over a long period of time; the number of errors becomes frighteningly astronomical. For these reasons, we recommend you always use double-check transcription methods for human transcription and that you regularly check machine transcription for accuracy. If you are printing on pre-printed forms, we also suggest regularly checking alignment to avoid any shifting of text.

5.9 Release of Results

5.9.1 General

The laboratory shall establish documented procedures for the release of examination results, including details of who may release results and to whom.

The procedures shall ensure that the following conditions are met:

a) When the quality of the primary sample received is unsuitable for examination or could have compromised the results, this is indicated on the report;
b) When examination results fall within established "alert" or "critical" intervals:
   - A physician (or other authorized health professional) is notified immediately [this includes results received on samples sent to referral laboratories for examination (see 4.5)];
   - Records are maintained of actions taken that document date, time, responsible laboratory staff member, person notified and examination results conveyed, and any difficulties encountered in notifications;
c) Results are legible, without mistakes in transcription, and reported to person(s) authorized to receive and use the information;
d) When results are transmitted as an interim report, the final report is always forwarded to the requester;
e) There are processes for ensuring that results distributed by telephone or electronic means reach only authorized recipients. Results provided orally shall be followed by a written report. There shall be a record of all oral results provided.

NOTE 1: For the results of some examinations (e.g., certain genetic or infectious disease examinations), special counseling may be needed. The laboratory should endeavor to see that results with serious implication are not communicated directly to the patient without the opportunity for adequate counseling.

NOTE 2: Results of laboratory examinations that have been separated from all patient identification may be used for such purpose as epidemiology, demography or other statistical analyses. See also 4.9.

REMARKS

The release of results is another important stage in the testing process where critical errors may occur. Common errors include:

a) Releasing results prior to QC review
b) Releasing results with out-of-range QC
c) Releasing results with obvious nonsense values
d) Releasing illegible results
e) Releasing results that, based on the test performed and clinical information, should be re-run for confirmation
f) Releasing results when the specimen did not meet criteria and the report contains no notification of this
g) Releasing results routinely when your Panic Value Policy requires immediate client notification
h) Releasing results without regard to privacy requirements
i) Releasing results without regard to counseling recommendation requirements
j) Releasing corrected reports that are not clearly identified as such
k) Releasing reports with missing data
l) Releasing reports with missing or inaccurate reference ranges

Identifying and correcting these kinds of problems can only be done if you ensure two things. First, does the person releasing the results have proper qualifications? And second, does the person releasing the results have knowledge about the laboratory's requirements and procedures?

Panic values represent a lab's biggest opportunity to positively impact patient cases. The speed and method for treating panic values will largely define your laboratory's value proposition, the quality of your relationship with clients, and perhaps even your overall economic sustainability. There is a problem, though. In our systemized and mechanized approach to operating clinical laboratories, we often tend to avoid processes that interrupt the routine workflow. So, it is interesting that the single biggest thing a laboratory absolutely must do right—reporting panic values—requires a complete break from routine. Since panic values require you to act fast and decisively, you must deal directly with clients—something potentially far from routine.

There are many ways to treat panic values. One way can be found in the sample policies and procedures for this FOS. We highly recommend that you regard panic values as opportunities to demonstrate value and cement quality relationships with your clients.

5.9.2 Automated Selection and Reporting of Results

If the laboratory implements a system for automated selection and reporting of results, it shall establish a documented procedure to ensure that:

a) The criteria for automated selection and reporting are defined, approved, readily available and understood by the staff;

   NOTE: Items for consideration when implementing automated selection and reporting include changes from previous patient values that require review and values that require intervention by laboratory personnel, such as absurd, unlikely or critical values.

b) The criteria are validated for proper functioning before use and verified after changes to the system that might affect their functioning;
c) There is a process for indicating the presence of sample interferences (e.g., hemolysis, icterus, lipemia) that may alter the results of the examination;
d) There is a process for incorporating analytical warning messages from the instruments into the automated selection and reporting criteria, when appropriate;

e) Results selected for automated reporting shall be identified at the time of review before release and include date and time selection;
f) There is a process for rapid suspension of automated selection and reporting.

REMARKS

In today's modern clinical laboratory, auto-verification systems are a reality, and they can be a useful tool. The biggest mistake labs make, however, is overreliance on those who produce and sell the software. These people are not typically laboratory scientists, and it is not their responsibility for lab results to be properly reported. They often don't understand the potentially life-threatening implications of releasing inaccurate results. As said earlier, such final responsibility lays solely with the laboratory and ultimately the laboratory director

At the same time, lab staff are hardly computer software engineers, so what can you do to ensure the auto-verification systems work? The answer is simple:

a) Test all parameters before placing a system into service
b) Re-test all parameters on a regular basis
c) Re-test all parameters after a software update or after any changes that may impact the data transmission process
d) Test your process to suspend reporting results when certain criteria are met

This may sound complicated, but it is not. All you need to do is create some dummy patient charts that include all potential resulting errors (i.e., absurd, unlikely and critical values; unit errors; decimal placement errors; all results requiring formulary calculations; lack of patient identification, values that exceed your delta check flags, etc.). Then, compare these results with a confirmed list of all possible errors you have entered into your fictionalized reports.

5.9.3 Revised Reports

When an original report is revised, there shall be written instructions regarding the revision so that:

a) The revised report is clearly identified as a revision and includes reference to the date and patient's identity in the original report;
b) The user is made aware of the revision;
c) The revised record shows the time and date of the change and the name of the person responsible for the change;
d) The original report entries remain in the record when revisions are made.

Results that have been made available for clinical decision-making and revised shall be retained in subsequent cumulative reports and clearly identified as having been revised.

When the reporting system cannot capture amendments, changes or alterations, a record of such shall be kept.

REMARKS

Multiple copies of the same report can cause confusion and inaccurate diagnosis, and, in some cases, lead to poor treatment decisions. Usually such problems occur when an initial incomplete report gets issued while awaiting the results of assays with prolonged turnaround times. Other causes include corrected reports. In our opinion, the best policy is to maintain all versions of reports, clearly marking the final or corrected report as such and highlighting newly added results or changes. A problem does exist here in that some LIS require that these steps be done manually. Also, some LIS have a specific way that corrected reports are displayed. This is perfectly acceptable as long as all the ISO 15189 requirements are met.

The reason why corrected/revised reports should bear the name of the editor(s) and time of correction/revision is that these reports can breed confusion in both the lab and with the client. Having names and times listed ensures that these questions are quickly and easily resolved. A time stamp to all revised versions helps to identify which version is the latest.

If your LIS cannot handle the functions mentioned above, you either will need to develop a manual workaround or find a different LIS provider. Work with your vendor to find a solution. It is likely that you are not their only customer who has to meet these requirements.

Why being in compliance with this FOS is important:

The patient report is your ultimate end product. The report (along with your customer service and contact) is the most visible part of your laboratory to your clients. Problems such as errors in your patient reports, unclear reports, report formats that are difficult to follow, difficulty in identifying the most current report, and correct results in a corrected reported will all be noticed by customers and can lead to incorrect diagnoses and patient harm.

Failing to quickly identify and report panic values can have a major impact on patient care. Problems with auto-verification systems can reproduce unnoticed reporting errors repeatedly and over long periods of time.

Materials Included In This FOS
• Reviewing and Reporting Results Policies and Procedures
• Test Report Criteria
• Test Report Form
• Acceptance Criteria for Release of Results
• List of Parameters Used for Validation of Auto-verification
• List of Critical Values
• Critical Value Log

FOS: Records Control / ISO 4.13

4.13 Control of Records

The laboratory shall have a documented procedure for identification, collection, indexing, access, storage, maintenance, amendment, and safe disposal of quality and technical records.

Records shall be created concurrently with performance of each activity that affects the quality of the examination.

NOTE 1: Records can be in any form or type of medium providing they are readily accessible and protected from unauthorized alterations.

The date and, where relevant, the time of amendments to records shall be captured along with the identity of personnel making the amendments (see 5.8.6).

The laboratory shall define the time period that various records—pertaining to the quality management system, including pre-examination, examination and post-examination processes—are retained. The length of time that records are retained may vary; however, reported results shall be retrievable for as long as medically relevant or as required by regulation.

NOTE 2: Legal liability concerns regarding certain types of procedures (e.g., histology examinations, genetic examinations, pediatric examinations) may require the retention of certain records for much longer than other records.

Facilities shall provide a suitable environment for storage of records to prevent damage, deterioration, loss or unauthorized access (see 5.2.6).

NOTE 3: For some records, especially those stored electronically, the safest storage may be on secure media and at an offsite location (see 5.9.4).

Records shall include, at least, the following:

a) Supplier selection and performance, and changes to the approved supplier;
b) Staff qualifications, training and competency records;

c) Requests for examinations;
d) Records of receipts of samples in the laboratory;
e) Information on reagents and materials used for examinations (e.g., lot documentation, certificates of supplies, package inserts);
f) Laboratory work books or work sheets;
g) Instrument printouts and retained data and information;
h) Examination results and reports;
i) Instrument maintenance records, including internal and external calibration records;
j) Calibration function and conversion factors;
k) Quality control record;
l) Incident records and action taken;
m) Accident records and action taken;
n) Risk management records;
o) Nonconformities identified and immediate or corrective action taken;
p) Preventative action taken;
q) Complaints and action taken;
r) Records of internal and external audits;
s) Inter-laboratory comparisons of examination results;
t) Records of quality improvement activities;
u) Minutes of meetings that record decisions made about the laboratory's quality management activities;
v) Records of management reviews.

All of these quality and technical records shall be made available for laboratory management review (see 4.15).

REMARKS

Laboratory records must be maintained for certain periods of time, depending on what the laboratory record is referring to. Below is a general guideline for maintaining laboratory records. Since it is not an all-inclusive list, it is best to check with your local laws and regulations about specific requirements for maintaining records and follow the more stringent requirement.

Type of Record	Period of Retention
General Laboratory Records	
Accession log records	2 years
Maintenance/instrument maintenance records	2 years
Quality control records	2 years
Surgical Pathology Records (including bone marrow)	
Reports	10 years
Cytology Records	
Reports	10 years
Non-Forensic Autopsy Records	
Reports	10 years
Forensic Autopsy Records	
Reports	Indefinitely
Gross photographs/negatives	Indefinitely
Accession log records	Indefinitely
Clinical Pathology Records	
Patient test records	2 years
Cytogenetics Records	
Final reports	20 years
Diagnostic images (digitized or negatives)	20 years
Blood Bank Records	
Donor records	10 years
Patient records	10 years
Records of employee signatures, initials, and identification codes	10 years
Quality control records	5 years
Records of indefinitely deferred donors, permanently deferred donors or donors placed under surveillance for the recipient's protection (e.g., those donors that are Hepatitis B Core positive once, donors implicated in a hepatitis positive recipient)	Indefinitely

Note that this FOS is found in each technical department as well and should allow you to separately manage records related to each department. The general rules (e.g., retention time), however, should be kept consistent. If your laboratory is on the smaller side, or if you choose to handle all laboratory records control within the QMS department, you can shift responsibility for some or all of the individual department's Record Control FOS requirements to the QMS department, so that this department will be solely responsible for managing this FOS.

Records indicated within this FOS may include those retained in other LEAP departments such as Personnel, Laboratory Director, Sample Collection, and all technical departments.

Why being in compliance with this FOS is important:

Maintaining laboratory records allows you to retrospectively look at the functioning of your laboratory at any time. You can trace today's problems back to the past to see if these recently recognized issues impacted past patient outcomes and enact remedies, if possible. Quality laboratory records also allow you to protect the laboratory if challenged by a user or in legal situations. And, of course, the maintenance of these records will be paramount to you maintaining your accreditation or certification status.

Materials Included In This FOS
• Records Control Policies and Procedures
• Laboratory Records Conformity Checklist
• Records Log

FOS: Quality Control / ISO 5.6, 5.6.1, 5.6.2, 5.6.2.1, 5.6.2.2, 5.6.2.3

5.6 Ensuring Quality of Examination Results

5.6.1 General

The laboratory shall ensure the quality of examinations by performing them under defined conditions.

Appropriate pre- and post-examination processes shall be implemented (see 4.14.7, 5.4, 5.7 and 5.8).

The laboratory shall not fabricate any results.

REMARKS

Most trained lab technicians will be familiar with quality control (QC). Having said that, let's examine the concept of "fabricating results" mentioned in 5.6.1 above. As we all know and surely agree, constructing false patient test results is one of the most horrendous acts a laboratory can commit. *BUT, it does happen.* There are hundreds of cases of "sink testing" reported annually in the United States alone. As you can imagine, the consequences are devastating for patient care (and for the offending technologists as well since they may face criminal action if discovered—possibly even as accessory to murder).

Monitoring for "sink testing" on larger scales can be done simply enough; just calculate average reagent usage by the number of tests reported and investigate any abnormalities.

Fabricating quality control results is also harmful. Of course, everyone wants to be proud of his/her QC results, but false reporting hurts everyone. One small example of how this might happen is a result that falls out of range; the test then gets re-run with a proper range but with the original poor result going unrecorded. This would constitute a fabricated result. If perfect QC results are due to the re-running of controls until one comes into range and not recording the out-of-range results, that is *not* QC.

Finally, everyone must understand that fabricating QC results can be even more damaging than "sink testing" single patient samples. It destroys the integrity of the process and can thus affect large numbers of patient results.

5.6.2 Quality Control

5.6.2.1 General

The laboratory shall design quality control procedures that verify the attainment of the intended quality of results.

NOTE: In several countries, quality control, as referred to in this subclause, is also named "internal quality control".

REMARKS

There are vast resources available that discuss internal quality control; therefore, we will not labor the point except briefly to bring up "clinical relevancy". The truth is we can become obsessed with refining quality control—and why not? It is at the core of what we do, and we should take pride in doing the best we can. If so, we cannot ignore the concept of "diminishing returns". For example, if you have an assay running with two standard deviations and you have evaluated this to satisfy the precision necessary for clinical interpretation, is there any value in expending resources to drive the standard deviation to 1.0? Beyond academic curiosity, the answer is probably no. As with all things under ISO, the degree of precision needed is dictated by the needs of the user. In the case of medical testing, this is largely driven by clinical utility.

This brings us to another point: blanket quality control rules. Some labs, for example, arbitrarily determine Coefficient of Variation (CV) and Standard Deviation (SD), and these are made applicable across all testing methods. Instead, we recommend you evaluate each testing method and then answer the question: what is the clinical tolerance? In some cases, a CV of 3.0 could be fine. In other situations, you will need to work hard to improve your QC so you can satisfy your user and clinical relevancy requirements.

Quality control has several defined rule sets. Perhaps the most widely used are the Westgard Rules, which are a set of rules that can be applied separately to each test based on clinical risk and other factors. We encourage your lab to examine the Westgard Rules and see if implementing them for particular tests is appropriate. If you are a CAP-accredited laboratory, you will need to institute IQCP rules for each test that is undergoing QC at a frequency less than what CAP or CLIA allows. This is required even if that lower frequency for QC is permitted by the test manufacturer. Under IQCP, you must establish QC frequency for each assay based on risk factors.

Lastly, there are a multitude of software products to help you record, analyze, and report quality control results as well as with auto-verification programs. While these can all be outstanding tools, they are only as good as the data reviewing process and how the lab staff use it.

5.6.2.2 Quality Control Materials

The laboratory shall use quality control materials that react to the examining system in a manner as close as possible to patient samples.

Quality control materials shall be periodically examined with a frequency that is based on the stability of the procedure and the risk of harm to the patient from an erroneous result.

NOTE 1: The laboratory should choose concentrations of control materials, wherever possible, especially at or near clinical decision values, which ensure the validity of decisions made.

NOTE 2: Use of independent third party control materials should be considered, either instead of or in addition to any control materials supplied by the reagent or instrument manufacturer.

REMARKS

There are several ways to source quality control materials. These include: a) controls purchased through a test vendor, either as part of a kit or separately; b) third party commercial controls; and c) validated pooled specimens.

Increasingly, the most common controls used in many countries are those included in commercial kits. These controls are often optimized for the particular kit, so you tend not to get any surprises. But many feel, like an audit with no findings, that optimized, vendor supplied controls do not really test the system. They feel that third party controls are more academically honest and reveal problems that would not come to light with a manufacturer's control material.

Using pooled specimens can be seen as an economic option for controls because your cost of the control material is essentially free in the form of excess patient sample. But these seemingly economic options can be deceiving when you look at the time and effort required to validate and verify these controls. Especially problematic can be attempts at providing control values covering the entire reportable range. It is for these reasons that, in many places, pooled controls are falling out of favor versus commercially available systems that come pre-validated and cover an appropriate spectrum of results.

There is something to note on control materials that can be important, especially with third party controls or pooled specimens. Many times, these controls may contain stabilizers and preservatives to extend their useful shelf life. These substances may interfere with some assay systems, such as the matrix effect seen with dry-chemistry. You always need to remember that controls are, by definition, different than patient samples due to added stabilizers, and this needs to be considered when troubleshooting out-of-range control results.

5.6.2.3 Quality Control Data

The laboratory shall have a procedure to prevent the release of patient results in the event of quality control failure.

When the quality control rules are violated and indicate that examination results are likely to contain clinically significant errors, the results shall be rejected and relevant patient samples re-examined after the error condition has been corrected and within-specification performance is verified. The laboratory shall also evaluate the results from patient samples that were examined after the last successful quality control event.

Quality control data shall be reviewed at regular intervals to detect trends in examination performance that may indicate problems in the examination system. When such trends are noted, preventative actions shall be taken and recorded.

NOTE: Statistical and non-statistical techniques for process control should be used wherever possible to continuously monitor examination system performance.

REMARKS

A complete discussion of evaluating quality control results is beyond the scope of this book. However, there are some important things to keep in mind. First, you need to establish acceptable QC ranges based on risk. Second, you need to evaluate control data before reporting results. And, lastly, if you are using an auto-verification system, it is essential to test this system regularly to ensure that results are not reported with out-of-range controls. The best way to do this is to purposely include control materials you know will be out-of-range and determine if your auto-verification system flags this prior to reporting results.

Why being in compliance with this FOS is important:

Falsifying results could kill people, land the fabricator in jail, and cause civil and criminal penalties for the laboratory and its director. Quality control materials that only evaluate a part of the reportable range will leave many results essentially non-controlled. Using inappropriate control materials will cause you to repeat results and spend a great deal of time troubleshooting. And lastly, not evaluating results properly is tantamount to doing no quality control at all. All of these things can lead to baked-in errors that can impact the care of thousands of patients.

Materials Included In This FOS
• Quality Control Policies and Procedures
• Standard Quality Control Document

FOS: Comparability of Results / ISO 5.6.4

5.6.4 Comparability of Examination Results

There shall be a defined means of comparing procedures, equipment and methods used and establishing the comparability of results for patient samples throughout the clinically appropriate intervals. This is applicable to the same of different procedures, equipment, different sites, or all of these.

NOTE: In the particular case of measurement results that are metrological comparability providing that calibrators are commutable.

The laboratory shall notify users of any differences in comparability of results and discuss any implications for clinical practice when measuring systems provide different measurement intervals for the same measure (e.g., glucose) and when examination methods are changed.

The laboratory shall document, record and, as appropriate, expeditiously act upon results from the comparison performed. Problems or deficiencies identified shall be acted upon and records of actions retained.

REMARKS

Many laboratories have more than one instrument or method that can perform the same testing. Whether it is the same make/model, a different instrument altogether, or a manual method, you must make sure that patient results for analytes correlate across all like testing. This is also true if your laboratory performs testing sent out to reference laboratories within your ISO scope of accreditation. These analytes must be correlated also.

Correlations must be performed according to the laboratory's written policies and regulatory requirements. Many laboratories that fall under CAP regulations must perform correlation testing twice a year. The following must be specified by the laboratory director prior to the correlation being performed:

a) The number of specimens to be tested for the correlation:
   Many laboratories perform correlations using twenty (20) samples. You should always follow your regulatory agency's requirements.

b) The cutoff for correlation to be considered acceptable:
   Once again, you should follow your regulatory agency's requirements.
c) Actions to take if there is a lack of correlation

For tests that are sent to referral laboratories, the laboratory must clarify to users that the testing is going to be done at referral laboratories and must also indicate this on their reports. The comparability criteria will not apply for these tests if, and only if, the laboratory has a method to qualify, evaluate, and monitor referral laboratories. Note that referral laboratories may have different ranges from the ones used in your laboratory and may change or alter their ranges over time.

One area to watch carefully is if you have a stat lab separate from the main lab. Significant differences in results can create a baked-in repeatable error (bias or systematic error) in many patients and for extended periods of times.

Why being in compliance with this FOS is important:

If you have multiple systems testing the same analyte and they are delivering different results that are clinically significant, it can lead to a wrong diagnosis. In case a clinician is using a serial testing result and the results are different (delta), it can create the impression of a shift in clinical presentation that is inaccurate, and may result in inaccurate dosing changes or even unnecessary diagnostic procedures, hospitalization, and/or surgery. It can also be a source of measurement uncertainty, and the variability needs to be taken into account when calculating measurement uncertainty.

Materials Included In This FOS
• Comparability of Results Policies and Procedures
• Comparability of Results Log

FOS: Risk Management / ISO 4.14.6

4.14.6 Risk Management

The laboratory shall evaluate the impact of work processes and potential failures on examination results as they affect patient safety, and shall modify processes to reduce or eliminate the identified risks and document decisions and actions taken.

REMARKS

Within the world of ISO, the definition of risk is a random event that has a negative impact (as defined in ISO 15190). There are two components to risk: the probability of occurrence of harm, and the severity of that harm. Laboratory risk management involves the assessment of both these components and applying the risk assessment into prioritization of QMS activities and into the performance of these activities.

There are a number of tools available to help with risk assessment and management: process mapping, fishbone diagrams, and risk grading systems. Our advice is to keep things simple. Use the tools that are most helpful or that you are most familiar with to analyze risk. Risk management is best as a team where you have the diversity of inputs and opinions to address issues and find solutions.

To comply with this standard, first and foremost you need to be vigilant. Look for problems everywhere at all times. To be effective, this vigilance needs to be instilled in everyone at all levels of the laboratory. As 4.14.6 largely depends on Nonconformities (4.9, 4.10, 4.11) and Quality Indicators (4.14.7), these FOSs are included in each technical department as well.

There are two kinds of risk that require management. First are problems that are already "symptomatic," that is, the results of the problem are already causing harm, and these should be dealt with immediately. Note that the objective of having a Risk Management Program is to identify and adopt measure that will either solve or prevent risks prior to them becoming "symptomatic" (i.e., before harm is caused).

Issues that can potentially impact patient safety are numerous and occur at all levels. Examples of risks for each stage include:

Pre-examination

a. Failure by the clinician to collect a proper sample
b. Failure associated to samples adhering to environmental or maximum time-to-assay standards
c. Excessive lipemia, hemolysis, or icteric samples
d. Malfunctions of refrigerators containing patient samples prior to assays being performed
e. Failure to collect patient demographic information such as age, gender, and clinical conditions which help identify samples and may be relevant to test results

Examination

a. Failure to review quality control prior to release of results and discovering post-fact that the results were not within range
b. Notification by reagent manufacturers concerning a recalled reagent lot you have already reported results from
c. Discovery of a carry-over problem in your system
d. Use of glassware with excess detergent residue
e. Problem employee reporting results without actually performing the tests

Post-examination

a. Transcription error(s) on patient reports
b. Wrong interpretation of test data/results by clinicians
c. Reporting results outside established turnaround time guidelines
d. Mistaking unit of measure noted on patient reports
e. Failure to include age and/or gender in patient reportable assays impacted by these factors

In all cases, the quality assurance department and laboratory director must be notified immediately so that the situation can be dealt with transparently and quickly. The primary objective is *not* to save face with the client. Instead, the goal is to focus solely on the patient: how best to mitigate the problem and decrease morbidity/mortality that might have resulted from such errors.

Identifying a problem and fixing it is typically how these issues get handled. The objective of 4.14.6 is to get the laboratory to proactively identify such risk factors prior to it becoming symptomatic and implement preventative measures and not only corrective measures. Periodic, system-wide analysis of your processes is one way of mitigating and managing risk. We strongly recommend that you include the entire staff in this process and encourage and reward staff members who identify possible risk factors and seek proactive solutions. When these issues are identified, they need to become agenda items for quality meetings so that they can be considered potential quality objectives and/or indicators.

Note that risk management reviews can be combined with internal audits or performed separately. Obviously, an independent review of risk management allows more focus and may be more effective. The results of your risk management activities must also be an input into your management reviews (4.15.2 (e)).

Risk management can involve issues outside of test results and patient safety. There are risks associated with employee safety (e.g., chemical and biological hazards) and legal risks (e.g., storing records for longer than the minimum necessary or longer than required by laboratory policy).

Lastly, risk assessment and management has become a crucial element in determining frequency of QC. The development of an Individual Quality Control Plan (IQCP) may be required when a laboratory departs from daily external QC requirements. These plans include an evaluation of risks associated to not performing daily QC with the level of harm that could result from inaccurate testing to determine the optimum frequency of running quality controls. This may be required, even if your vendor has gotten approval for less frequent quality control. You should refer to your local regulations to see if IQCP is required in your area.

Why being in compliance with this FOS is important:

There are a number of overarching reasons why risk management is important to the laboratory. First, there is the overall moral duty that the laboratory management has to reduce risk to its employees and patients. The implications of not managing risk can have very serious consequences. If unmanaged risks occur, it can seriously weaken the confidence that other areas of the hospital or the public has in the laboratory.

Also, problems in the laboratory tend to be repetitive rather than one-off occurrences. In other words, laboratory problems have a tendency to be "baked-in" and affect many patients over long periods of time. There are noteworthy examples of laboratories reporting out hundreds of thousands or even millions of erroneous results over periods lasting decades. This is why laboratories frequently require a QMS system separate from other hospital departments, and we all need to be on the lookout for these kinds of errors and actively seek to find and fix them.

Risk management not only solves existing problems, but, in its purest state, allows the laboratory to prioritize quality activities and concentrate on tackling issues that pose the greatest risk.

Materials Included In This FOS
• Risk Management Policies and Procedures
• Guidance on Risk Assessment
• Preventative Action Plan
• Quality Meeting Minutes

FOS: Nonconformities / ISO 4.9, 4.10, 4.11

4.9 Identification and Control of Nonconformities

The laboratory shall have a documented procedure to identify and manage nonconformities in any aspect of the quality management system, including pre-examination, examination, or post-examination processes.

The procedure shall ensure that:

a) The responsibilities and authorities for handling nonconformities are designated;
b) The immediate actions to be taken are defined;
c) The extent of the nonconformity is determined;
d) Examinations are halted and reports withheld as necessary;
e) The medical significance of any nonconforming examination is considered and, where applicable, the requesting clinician or authorized individual responsible for using the results is informed;
f) The results of any nonconformities or potentially nonconforming examinations already are recalled or appropriately identified, as necessary;
g) The responsibility for authorization of the resumption of examinations is defined;
h) Each episode of nonconformity is documented and recorded, with these records being reviewed at regular specified intervals to detect trends and initiate corrective action.

NOTE: Nonconforming examinations or activities occur in many different areas and can be identified in many different ways, including clinician complaints, internal quality control indications, instrument calibrations, checking for consumable materials, inter-laboratory comparison, staff comments, reporting and certificate checking, laboratory management reviews, and internal and external audits.

When it is determined that nonconformities in pre-examination, examination and post-examination processes could recur or that there is doubt about the laboratory's compliance with its own procedures, the laboratory shall take action to identify, document and eliminate the cause(s).

Corrective action to be taken shall be determined and documented (see 4.10).

4.10 Corrective Action

The laboratory shall take corrective action to eliminate the cause(s) of nonconformities.

Corrective actions shall be appropriate to the effects of the nonconformities encountered.

The laboratory shall have documented procedures for:

a) Reviewing nonconformities;
b) Determining the root cause of nonconformities;
c) Evaluating the need for corrective action to ensure that nonconformities do not recur;
d) Determining and implementing corrective action needed;
e) Recording the results of corrective action taken (see 4.14.5);
f) Reviewing the effectiveness of the corrective action taken (see 4.15).

NOTE: Action taken at the time of the nonconformity to mitigate its immediate effects is considered 'immediate' action. Only action taken to remove the root cause of the problem that is causing the nonconformities is considered 'corrective action'.

4.11 Preventative Action

The laboratory shall determine action to eliminate the causes of potential nonconformities in order to prevent their occurrence. Preventative actions shall be appropriate to the effects of the potential problems.

The laboratory shall have a documented procedure for:

a) Reviewing laboratory data and information to determine where potential nonconformities exist;
b) Determining the root cause(s) of potential nonconformities;
c) Evaluating the need for preventative action to prevent the occurrence of nonconformities;

d) Determining and implementing preventative action needed;
e) Recording the results of preventative action taken (see 4.13);
f) Reviewing the effectiveness of the preventative action taken.

NOTE: Preventative action is a proactive process for identifying opportunities for improvement rather than a reaction to the identification of a problem or complaints (i.e., nonconformities). In addition to review of the operation procedures, preventative action might involve analysis of data, including trend and risk analyses and external quality assessment (proficiency testing).

REMARKS

Basically, what is being asked of you here is:

a) To adhere to your own policies and procedures
b) To have ways of ensuring you are adhering to your own policies and procedures
c) When you discover you are not complying with your own policies and procedures, to have some documented way of returning to compliance
d) When you find you are not complying with your own policies and procedures, determine if damage had been done and perform corrective action, if necessary
e) Identify ways to proactively make sure you do not violate your own policies and procedures

You can identify nonconformities the hard or easy way. The hard way refers to situations where some kind of nonconformity causes harm, and you must deal with, not only correcting the nonconformity, but the consequences of the harm as well. The easy way would be identifying a nonconformity during an internal or external audit. There is also a best way—remaining in compliance with your policies and procedures at all times to minimize the occurrence of nonconformities.

The goal of staying in constant compliance is obvious; at the same time, it can be challenging. Luckily, you are a LEAP user. If you set up your QMS Maintenance properly and your task managers respond to email reminders and/or vigilantly monitor their personal My Tasks page, you can stay in compliance 24/7.

Why being in compliance with this FOS is important:

All too often, laboratory errors are not single failures to follow procedures. Rather, they tend to get baked into the system with inadequate procedures or systematic practices of not following them. For example, if your normal range is shifted and this shift was not recognized when it occurred, the results for all patients can get reported in error for extended periods of time. Even something as simple as a single non-calibrated pipette can reverberate throughout your laboratory in unpredictable ways. Identifying nonconformities quickly and dealing with them effectively is the hallmark of every quality laboratory. Your ability to do this well will impact your productivity, your staff, and the quality of patient care.

Materials Included In This FOS
• Nonconformities Policies and Procedures
• Nonconformity Event Reporting Form
• Nonconformity Event Investigation Log

FOS: Management Review / ISO 4.15, 4.15.1, 4.15.2, 4.15.3, 4.15.4

4.15 Management Review

4.15.1 General

Laboratory management shall review the quality management system at planned intervals to ensure its continuing suitability, adequacy and effectiveness and support of patient care.

4.15.2 Review Input

The input to management review shall include information from the results of evaluations of at least the following:

a) The periodic review of requests, and suitability of procedures and sample requirements (see 4.14.2);
b) Assessment of user feedback (see 4.14.3);
c) Staff suggestion (see 4.14.4);
d) Internal audits (see 4.14.5);
e) Risk management (see 4.14.6);
f) Use of quality indicators (see 4.14.7);
g) Reviews by external organizations (see 4.14.8);
h) Results of participation in inter-laboratory comparison program (PT. EQA) (see 5.6.3);
i) Monitoring and resolution of complaints (see 4.8);
j) Performance of suppliers (see 4.6);
k) Identification and control of nonconformities (see 4.9);
l) Results of continual improvement (see 4.12) including current status of corrective actions (see 4.10) and preventative actions (see 4.11);
m) Follow-up actions from previous management reviews;
n) Changes in the volume and scope of work, personnel, and premises that could affect the quality management system;
o) Recommendations for improvement, including technical requirements.

REMARKS

Doing a management review for each of the above items looks daunting, and it certainly can be. The best way for you to manage the review is through strict compliance with all LEAP-generated management tasks. Make sure and assign responsible maintenance task managers and monitor your LEAP Maintenance Dashboard.

If you choose not to use LEAP for maintenance purposes, you will need to carefully incorporate these items into your quality meetings and take meticulous notes. You must also be prepared to locate these notes during an inspection and make sure you keep software copies and use keyword searches. Keywords are far more useful if you standardize lab vocabulary. Unless your staff share terminology, one person's "External Quality Control" may be labeled "CAP Survey" by someone else.

In short, the best advice from us is to use LEAP maintenance features.

4.15.3 Review Activities

The review shall analyze the input information for cause of nonconformities, trends and patterns that indicate process problems.

This review shall include assessing these opportunities for improvement and the need for changes to the quality management system, including the quality policy and quality objectives.

The quality and appropriateness of the laboratory's contribution to patient care shall, to the extent possible, also be objectively evaluated.

REMARKS

At the risk of sounding like a broken record, we once again recommend that you use LEAP maintenance features effectively—in other words, ensure that your personnel reviews each and every process with a highly critical eye.

Things change over time, so make sure you analyze all the changes, regardless of whether the changes are to facilities, personnel, instrumentation, or any new knowledge/information you and/or your staff may have acquired.

If you choose not to use LEAP, stock up on clipboards and checklists and ensure all of the necessary records are kept on a daily, weekly, monthly, basis. You will have to be very organized and constantly monitor these, ensuring documentation of everything.

4.15.4 Review Output

The output from the management review shall be incorporated into a record that documents any decisions made and actions taken during management review to:

a) Improve the effectiveness of the quality management system and its processes;
b) Improve service to users;
c) Resources needed.

NOTE: The interval between management reviews should be no longer than twelve (12) months; however, shorter intervals should be adopted when a quality management system is being established.

Findings and actions arising from management reviews shall be recorded and reported to laboratory staff.

Laboratory management shall ensure that actions arising from management review are completed within a defined timeframe.

REMARKS

In your periodic reviews, you should carefully look at the changes that were made before and after the last review. In these reviews, you should include things that you have learned and then identify all changes made and make appropriate modifications. You should review the efficacy of management changes and determine if it solved the problem or made things worse.

It is also important to double-check everything and ensure that all stakeholders are notified about these changes. For items with broad implications, it is smart to include them as agenda items for quality meetings since they could potentially become future quality objectives or indicators. As usual, don't forget to document everything in the Quality Meeting Minutes Form and load this into LEAP MF for easy recapture, communication to staff, and use in internal/external audits.

Why being in compliance with this FOS is important:

QMS requires a great many activity streams to be monitored: nonconformities, internal/external audits, risk management, staffing issues, etc. The objective of the management review is to bring this all together and review everything in context and how it relates to other issues. Doing this right will give your laboratory the big picture.

Materials Included In This FOS
• Management Review Policies and Procedures
• Management Review Checklist
• Management Review Meeting Minutes

FOS: Validation & Verification of Examination Procedures / ISO 5.5, 5.5.1, 5.5.1.1, 5.5.1.2, 5.5.1.3, 5.5.1.4, 5.5.2

5.5 Examination Processes

5.5.1 Selection, Verification and Validation of Examination Procedures

5.5.1.1 General

The laboratory shall select examination procedures, which have been validated for their intended use.

The identity of persons performing activities in examination processes shall be recorded.

The specific requirements (performance specifications) for each examination procedure shall relate to the intended use of that examination.

NOTE: Preferred procedures are those specified in the instructions for use of *in vitro* medical devices or those that have been published in established/authoritative textbooks, peer-reviewed texts or journals, or in international consensus standards or guidelines, or in national or regional regulations.

5.5.1.2 Verification of Examination Procedures

Validated examination procedures used without modification shall be subject to independent verification by the laboratory before being introduced into routine use.

The laboratory shall obtain information from the manufacturer/method developer for confirming the performance characteristics of the procedure.

The independent verification by the laboratory shall confirm, through obtaining objective evidence (in the form of performance characteristics) that the performance claims for the examination procedure have been met. The performance claims for the examination procedure confirmed during the verification process shall be those relevant to the intended use of the examination results.

The laboratory shall document the procedure used for the verification and record results obtained. Staff with the appropriate authority shall review the verification results and record the review.

5.5.1.3 Validation of Examination Procedures

The laboratory shall validate examination procedures derived from the following sources:

a) Non-standard methods;
b) Laboratory designed or developed methods;
c) Standard methods used outside their intended scope;
d) Validated methods subsequently modified.

The validation shall be as extensive as is necessary and confirm, through the provision of objective evidence (in the form of performance characteristics), that the specific requirements for the intended use of the examination have been fulfilled.

NOTE: Performance characteristics of an examination procedure should include consideration of: measurement trueness; measurement accuracy; measurement precision including measurement repeatability and measurement intermediate precision; measurement uncertainty; analytical specificity including interfering substances, analytical sensitivity, detection limit and quantitation limit; measuring interval; diagnostic specificity; and diagnostic sensitivity.

The laboratory shall document the procedure used for the validation and record the results obtained. Staff with the appropriate authority shall review the validation and record the review.

When changes are made to a validated examination procedure, the influence of such changes shall be documented and, when appropriate, a new validation shall be carried out.

5.5.1.4 Measurement Uncertainty of Measured Quantity Values

The laboratory shall determine measurement uncertainty for each measurement procedure in the examination phase used to report measured quantity values on patients' samples.

The laboratory shall define the performance requirements for the measurement uncertainty of each measurement procedure and regularly review estimates of measurement uncertainty.

NOTE 1: The relevant uncertainties components are those associated with the actual measurement process, commencing with the presentation of the sample to the measurement procedure and ending with the output of the measure value.

NOTE 2: Measurement uncertainties may be calculated using quantity values obtained by the measurement of quality control materials under intermediate precision conditions that include as many routine changes as reasonably possible in the standard operation of a measurement procedure, e.g., changes of reagent and calibrator batches, different operators, scheduled instrument maintenance.

NOTE 3: Examples of the practical utility of measurement uncertainty estimates might include confirmation that patients' values meet quality goals set by the laboratory and meaningful comparison of a patient value with a previous value of the same type or with a clinical decision value.

The laboratory shall consider measurement uncertainty when interpreting measured quantity values.

Upon request, the laboratory shall make its estimates of measurement uncertainty available to laboratory users.

Where examinations include a measurement step but do not report a measured quantity value, the laboratory should calculate the uncertainty of the measurement step where its utility is assessing the reliability of the examination procedure or has influence on the reported result.

5.5.2 Biological Reference Intervals or Clinical Decision Values

The laboratory shall define the biological reference intervals or clinical decision values, document the basis for the reference intervals or decision values and communicate this information to the users.

When a particular biological reference interval or decision value is no longer relevant for the population served, appropriate changes shall be made and communicated to the users.

When the laboratory changes an examination procedure or pre-examination procedure, the laboratory shall review associated reference intervals and clinical decision values, as applicable.

REMARKS

The process of validation and verification is essential for ensuring examinations are performing to specification and providing users with information they need to accurately diagnose and treat patients. In general terms, there are two kinds of validation and verification processes: a) kits that have been pre-validated by an external manufacturer; and b) assays that are made in your laboratory (Laboratory Developed Tests, or LDT). Kits that have been pre-validated by an external manufacturer for which you have deviated the process approved by that manufacturer must be treated as LDT.

If testing procedures are manufactured by another company and approved by a regulatory body (if required by local laws), the validation procedure (sometimes referred to as verification) needs to include the reagents as well as any other equipment or materials used in the examination process. While it is understood that manufacturers do their best to validate their products to their published specifications, they are ultimately not responsible for the welfare of patients. Therefore, in order to obtain and maintain accreditation, the laboratory itself is responsible for verifying that the assay systems are working to specification in your environment, with your equipment and with your personnel.

In case you are developing your own testing methodologies, the importance of validating and verifying those procedures prior to testing patients is even more important. If you choose to develop your own procedures (i.e., LDTs), for all intents and purposes, you will be required to take all steps required by a manufacturer of analytical systems. The methods vary depending upon technology and are beyond the scope of this document. However, most of the validation and verification procedures outlined in this document will apply.

The following is a list of validation and verification procedures which need to be taken for all assays prior to initiating patient testing:

a) Linearity and Analytical Measurement Range (AMR)/Dynamic Range
b) Precision (sometimes referred to as repeatability)
c) Accuracy
d) Correlation with Other Instruments or Methodologies
e) Interfering Substances Validation
f) Reportable Clinical Decision Values/Biological Reference Intervals
g) Measurement Uncertainty (MU)
h) Specimen Storage, Stability and Transportation Requirements
i) Dilution and Concentration Procedures (if applicable)

Simple examples of procedures have been included in this FOS, but please note that these procedures will vary depending upon the science and method of each examination and can be especially challenging in case of LDTs. Ensure that your thresholds for acceptability are established and documented before evaluating validation results, which should also be recorded. You are encouraged to consult CLSI guidelines.

Measurement Uncertainty (MU) is a relatively new concept for clinical laboratories and may be difficult to understand. You are encouraged to go to the following article for a complete and easy-to-understand explanation:

https://www.westgard.com/hitchhike-mu.htm

The laboratory director is ultimately responsible for approving these validations and authorizing their release for patient testing.

Why being in compliance with this FOS is important:

Validating and verifying your procedures both initially and after potentially impactful events can better assure the laboratory is not reporting aberrant results. It is noteworthy that these biases and aberrant results tend to be inherent in laboratory processes and may persist for long periods of time, impacting scores of patients, the reputation of the laboratory, and possible legal challenges.

Properly validating and verifying your procedures allows you to report results with confidence, knowing that you have confirmed, by all reasonable means, that the results reported are within your established tolerance limits. Remember, the laboratory is responsible for the quality of results, not the manufacturer of the instruments or reagent systems.

Materials Included In This FOS
• Validation and Verification of Examination Procedures Policies and Procedures
• Personnel Authorized to Confirm Validation and Verification Results
• Linearity and Analytical Measurement Range (AMR)/Dynamic Range Studies
• Linearity Calculation Worksheet
• Precision Studies
• Precision Calculation Worksheet
• Correlation Studies
• Interfering Substances Validation Studies
• Reportable Clinical Decision Values/Biological Reference Intervals Validation Studies
• Measurement Uncertainty (MU)

FOS: Quality Management Systems (QMS) / ISO 4.1.2.3, 4.1.2.4, 4.2, 4.2.1, 4.2.2.1, 4.2.2.2, 4.12

4.1.2.3 Quality Policy

Laboratory management shall define the intent of its quality management system in a quality policy.

Laboratory management shall ensure that the quality policy:

a) Is appropriate to the purpose of the organization;
b) Includes a commitment to good professional practice, examinations that are fit for intended use, compliance with the requirements of this International Standard, and continual improvement of the quality of laboratory services;
c) Provides a framework for establishing and reviewing quality objectives;
d) Is communicated and understood within the organization;
e) Is reviewed for continuing suitability.

REMARKS

Refer to the Laboratory Director Department FOS Management Commitment for what a quality policy can look like. Note that the quality policy should be drafted by the quality manager with input from the laboratory director and should demonstrate a clear understanding of the laboratory's operations, strengths, and weaknesses.

To ensure consistent and ongoing quality improvement, the quality process needs to have a proper framework in place as soon as possible. Key elements include: an empowered quality manager with a clear job description; periodic, documented quality meetings including monitoring of quality indicators; and documentation and review of sentinel events, among others.

The quality policy must regularly be reviewed and LEAP can help you do this through its Maintenance features.

4.1.2.4 Quality Objectives Planning

Laboratory management shall establish quality objectives, including those needed to meet the needs and requirements of the users, at relevant functions and levels within the organization. The quality objectives shall be measurable and consistent with the quality policy.

Laboratory management shall ensure that planning of the quality management system is carried out to meet the requirements (see 4.2) and the quality objectives.

Laboratory management shall ensure that the integrity of the quality management system is maintained when changes to the quality management system are planned and implemented.

REMARKS

Quality objectives = things you want to improve or monitor for acceptability.

These objectives can relate to quality control, safety, patient services, staff education, client education, optimizing instrumentation and/or reagent systems, as well as finding faster or more economic ways of doing lab functions.

For best results, quality objectives should have a clear target (or threshold for acceptability) and some way of tracking performance over time against your declared objectives.

Your management reviews should include a review of both the performance of the quality objectives and whether these objectives should be continued/discontinued or modified.

QMS needs to be a living system. Critically examining your quality objectives is essential for continued stability. If an objective is constantly being met, perhaps you need to allocate your limited quality resources someplace else. Also consider examining your thresholds for action. You may want to tighten your acceptability criteria so that all of your quality objectives represent a challenge to your current practices. Selection of quality objectives should be guided by your management reviews and, in particular, by your risk management.

Therefore, quality objectives may be continued for a while, even in light of continuous acceptable performance. You may be required to keep some for regulatory or accreditation purposes. If so, have a clear understanding of which objectives are required for what reason(s). Even those external requirements can change over time.

Please note that the quality objectives will be defined for the laboratory overall, and quality indicators will be created and monitored in accordance with these objectives. Indicators will be developed for the entire lab as well as for each individual department. The Quality Manager should work closely with each Department Manager to develop and monitor relevant indicators and ensure the objectives for the laboratory take the individual department issues into consideration.

4.2 Quality Management System

4.2.1 General Requirements

The laboratory shall establish, document, implement and maintain a quality management system and continually improve its effectiveness in accordance with the requirements of this International Standard.

The quality management system shall provide for the integration of all processes required to fulfill its quality policy and objectives and meet the needs and requirements of the users.

The laboratory shall:

a) Determine the processes needed for all the quality management system and ensure their application throughout the laboratory;
b) Determine the sequence and interaction of these processes;
c) Determine criteria and methods needed to ensure that both the operation and control of these processes are effective ;
d) Ensure the availability of resources and information necessary to support the operation and monitoring of these processes;
e) Monitor and evaluate these processes;
f) Implement actions necessary to achieve planned results and continual improvement of these processes.

4.2.2.1 General

The quality management system documentation shall include:

a) Statements of a quality policy (see 4.1.2.3) and quality objectives (see 4.1.2.4);
b) A quality manual (see 4.2.2.2);
c) Procedures and records required by this International Standard;
d) Documents and records (see 4.13) determined by the laboratory to ensure the effective planning, operation and control of its processes;
e) Copies of applicable regulations, standards and other normative documents.

NOTE: The documentation can be in any form or type of medium, providing it is readily accessible and protected from unauthorized changes and undue deterioration.

REMARKS

You will find templates and samples of most, if not all, of the documents listed above. You can use these and discuss with your LEAP QMS coach to help create a quality management system with appropriate documentation suitable for your laboratory. Remember, it is very important that you do what you say you are going to do and that everything is documented. If something is not written and/or recorded, it is the same as not doing it.

4.2.2.2 Quality Manual

The laboratory shall establish and maintain a quality manual that includes:

a) The quality policy (4.1.2.3) or makes reference to it;
b) A description of the scope of the quality management system;
c) A presentation of the organization and management structure of the laboratory and its place in any parent organization;
d) A description of roles and responsibilities of the laboratory management (including the laboratory director and quality manager) for ensuring compliance with this International Standard;

e) A description of the structure and relationships of the documentation used in the quality management system;
f) The documented policies established for the quality management system and reference to the managerial and technical activities that support them.

All laboratory staff shall have access to and be instructed on the use and application of the quality manual and the referenced documents.

REMARKS

The Quality Manual is your most important tool to map out your QMS journey. While your best quality manual is likely LEAP itself, some ISO inspectors may require you maintain a discrete manual.

While contemporary wisdom dictates that you create a Quality Manual *first*, prior to creating your systems, LEAP recommends the opposite approach. We recommend going through the process of building each element of your Quality Manual (i.e., FOS) and then copying and pasting these elements to create a discrete Quality Manual.

If you choose to have a separate Quality Manual outside of LEAP, you will need to remember to update it on a regular basis and ensure that any changes made when maintaining your QMS within LEAP and audits are being reflected accordingly.

4.12 Continual Improvement

The laboratory shall continually improve the effectiveness of the quality management systems, including the pre-examination, examination and post-examination processes, through the use of management reviews to compare the laboratory's actual performance in its evaluation activities, corrective actions and preventative actions with its intentions, as stated in the quality policy and quality objectives.

Action plans for improvement shall be developed, documented and implemented, as appropriate.

The effectiveness of the actions taken shall be determined through focused review or audit of the area concerned (see also 4.14.5).

Laboratory management shall ensure that the laboratory participates in continual improvement activities that encompass relevant areas and outcomes of patient care.

When continual improvement program identifies opportunities for improvement, laboratory management shall address them regardless of where they occur.

Laboratory management shall communicate to staff improvement plans and related goals.

REMARKS

At the heart of the statement immediately above is the idea that quality objectives are constantly evolving and that they are prioritized first by risk and then by projected benefit(s). For example, let's imagine that one of your quality objectives is to improve laboratory safety and the related quality indicator is baseline of 50 needle-sticks over the past twelve (12) months. In this example, "safety" would almost certainly be your top quality objective with "decreasing needle-sticks" as your top quality indicator. Please refer to Laboratory Director Department FOS Management Commitment and Quality Indicator for more details on each.

Think of building and maintaining Quality Management Systems (QMS) as a cascade of events. First, you have a quality policy to provide overall guidance. You then create quality objectives describing specific areas of desired improvement. This stage is then followed by creating specific, quantifiable quality indicators with defined performance thresholds to drive forward your objectives.

You also need to define specific procedures as to how you will perform the processes dictated by your quality policy and you will need to define the roles and responsibilities of those involved. You will need to ensure that you have allocated sufficient resources to monitoring, tracking, and improving quality.

You should evaluate quality objectives and indicators in terms of fixing a problem and in terms of improvement with this evaluation documented. Once these objectives and indicators are considered fulfilled or concluded, new objectives and indicators should be introduced to continuously challenge the laboratory. The Quality Manual ties everything together by providing an overall guidance plan that lays out the entire scheme, step-by-step and in detail.

Why being in compliance with this FOS is important:

Your Quality Management System (QMS) is what ties everything together. Failing to develop, maintain, and continuously improve this system and the details within likely means you fail to reap the benefits of all your hard work and are at increased risk of error which may in turn impact patient care.

Materials Included In This FOS
• Quality Management Systems (QMS) Policies and Procedures
• Quality Manual

FOS: Referral Laboratories / ISO 4.5, 4.5.1, 4.5.2

4.5 Examination by Referral Laboratories

4.5.1 Selecting and Evaluating Referral Laboratories and Consultants

The laboratory shall have a documented procedure for selecting and evaluating referral laboratories and consultants who provide opinions as well as interpretation for complex testing in any discipline.

The procedure shall ensure that the following are met:

a) The laboratory, with the advice of laboratory services where appropriate, is responsible for selecting the referral laboratory and referral consultants, monitoring the quality of performance and ensuring that the referral laboratories or referral consultants are competent to perform the requested examinations;
b) Arrangements with referral laboratories and consultants are reviewed and evaluated periodically to ensure that the relevant parts of this International Standard are met;
c) Records of such periodic reviews are maintained;
d) A register of all referral laboratories and consultants from whom opinions are sought is maintained;
e) Requests and results of all samples referred are kept for a pre-defined period.

REMARKS

Under ISO 15189, a laboratory can choose what testing is within its scope and what is not. The section of referral laboratory selection applies only to laboratories and testing that is within the laboratory's scope of accreditation. Therefore, if your laboratory sends out testing within its scope (either on a regular basis or as a back-up in case of overflow or downtime), then this standard applies. If all of the laboratory's referral testing is outside its ISO 15189 scope, then the requirements of referral testing are not strictly applicable. It is still best practice, however, to follow the standard for evaluation of referral testing even if it is not absolutely required.

The interpretation of this standard can also vary and requires an element of judgement. As case in point, imagine a procedure requiring a referral laboratory to be certified or accredited by a competent body (e.g., CAP rules for all CAP-accredited laboratories state that, when a second sample is sent to a referral lab, that lab must also be CAP-accredited). On the less onerous side, you could interpret this standard to mean any referral laboratory that is licensed by the government. On the opposite extreme, your procedure may demand your acceptance of referral labs would depend on that lab being ISO 15189-certified, CAP-accredited, and even be subject to a direct inspection by you. Judgement is, therefore, required as you need to determine your extent of requirements for a referral laboratory or consultant. Remember that whatever process and requirements you decide must be followed. Do not set the bar and process to high, or you may not be able to meet your own requirements.

Another factor to consider is the lab's history. If a laboratory is new, your procedures may call for an onsite inspection prior to entering an agreement. You can always do more than the minimum that your procedure requires, you just cannot do less. This also applies to separate laboratories within the same system or organization. Your selection and evaluation processes apply to all.

You must also consider the complexity of the testing being performed as well as the risk profile for inaccurate results. For example, if you are referring samples to a university lab and that test is very new and/or highly complex and/or the results of this testing could have a major impact on patient outcomes, part of your selection criteria may include interviewing the people managing the process. It is good to use your own risk management in assessing your quality requirements for referral laboratories as well as your own lab.

Regardless of your selection criteria and referral laboratory selection procedures, people and situations change within any lab. There may also be changes to your technology requirements based on the addition of new clients or clinical scope. For all these reasons, it is imperative that you review both the appropriateness of your referral lab/consultant selection criteria and the referral lab/consultant themselves. Generally, these reviews would happen annually but there is scope for flexibility. Reviews may be as simple as requesting a copy of the referral laboratory's accreditation or the consultant's qualifications.

Please note that a sample document with selection criteria is included in the Content Library for this FOS; however, this should only be used as a guide, and you are encouraged to examine and modify it according to your own needs. Do not be afraid to ask questions to your referral laboratories/consultants. If they are having problems with accuracy, experiencing transcription error, or do not meet your clinically required turnaround times, do not be shy about having a pointed discussion with this lab's representative. Finally, if they cannot fix the issues, shop around.

Do not let cost be your only consideration for selecting a referral laboratory. Ensure the choice is free from conflict of interest and do not succumb to pressure from external sources trying to dictate your laboratory selection. It must be the choice of the laboratory taking into account the needs of the users.

As discussed in 4.5.2, even when referring samples to another laboratory, it is your laboratory that is ultimately responsible for all results.

Finally, as a reminder, you may not send your external proficiency testing samples to a referral laboratory, even if that would be your normal procedure with clinical specimens (5.6.3).

4.5.2 Provisions of Examination Results

Unless otherwise specified in the agreement, the referring laboratory (and not the referral laboratory) shall be responsible for ensuring that examination results of the referral laboratory are provided to the person making the request.

When the referring laboratory prepares the report, it shall include all essential elements of the results reported by the referral laboratory or consultant, without alterations that could affect clinical interpretation. The report shall indicate which examinations were performed by a referral laboratory or consultant.

The author of any additional remarks shall clearly be identified.

Laboratories shall adopt the most appropriate means of reporting referral laboratory results, taking into account turnaround times, measurement accuracy, transcription processes and interpretive skill requirements. In cases where the correct interpretation and application of examination results needs collaboration between clinicians and specialists from both referring and referral laboratories, this process shall not be hindered by commercial or financial consideration.

REMARKS

When your laboratory refers samples to other labs, the bottom line is this: your laboratory remains ultimately responsible for all testing. Pre-analytically, it is your responsibility to ensure appropriate specimens are collected and provided under proper environmental conditions and that the referral laboratory/consultant has all necessary information. You also need to have confidence that your method of specimen transport to the referral laboratory (whether by them, you, or a third party) transports specimens with environmental stability. Finally, the referral laboratory needs any and all information required to complete the analytical processes and, in some cases, provide accurate post-analytical support.

One common problem is failing to provide adequate information to the referral laboratory/consultant. They need to know a patient's age, gender, and any clinical issues because well-run referral labs can and will issue life-saving panic value alerts based on this information.

Transcription errors are another source of post-analytical errors—which begs the question: if values are input manually, does your laboratory have error-checking protocols in place for duplicate entries?

Another key question would be: when interpretations are provided by a pathologist who is a consultant, what happens if the clinician has questions that only one person can answer and that person is not identified in the report?

You also need to make clear to your users which tests were performed by a referral laboratory and which laboratory reported those results. This can sometimes be difficult when you are using multiple laboratories, report out a portion of a particular report, use a distributive test system, or refer tests only when there is overflow or instrument downtime. As difficult as this sometimes can be, it is absolutely required that the user knows where each test was performed.

The provisions in this FOS are of vital importance to operating a quality lab, and they all too often get overlooked because these are not viewed to be the referral lab's responsibility. If you want to provide your clients with optimal service, you need to make it your responsibility, and the ISO standards require you to do so.

Why being in compliance with this FOS is important:

If your referral laboratories or consultants are giving inaccurate information, or your laboratory is not accurately transcribing data and associated guidance, this will negatively impact patient outcomes. On the positive side, policies that facilitate a collaborative and good relationship with your referral laboratories or consultants can increase your lab's ability to act effectively in emergent situations and even help you economically due to the ongoing monitoring and evaluation of business conditions and performance.

Materials Included In This FOS
• Referral Laboratories Policies and Procedures
• Referral Laboratory Checklist
• Consultant Competency Assessment Worksheet
• List of Approved Referral Laboratories and Consultants

TECHNICAL

FOS: Reagents & Consumables Management / ISO 5.3.2, 5.3.2.1, 5.3.2.2, 5.3.2.3, 5.3.2.4, 5.3.2.5, 5.3.2.7

5.3.2 Reagents and Consumables

5.3.2.1 General

The laboratory shall have a documented procedure for the reception, storage, acceptance testing and inventory management of reagents and consumables.

REMARKS

Reagents and consumables have a lifecycle. They are born and quality-assured in a factory, delivered to your laboratory, stocked in your inventory, put into service, utilized, and then discarded. Given that these items are process-driven, it is important to look at the entire lifecycle and consider three fundamental questions:

1. At each stage, what are the opportunities for reagents to become compromised?
2. Where in the reagent lifecycle can we best intervene to ensure they do not get compromised?
3. What steps can the laboratory take to ensure that only viable reagents are in use?

Key areas that need to be considered are: a) the manufacturer; b) distributors; c) delivery services; and d) the point of reception at the hospital and laboratory.

5.3.2.2 Reagents and Consumables – Reception and Storage

Where the laboratory is not the receiving facility, it shall verify that the receiving location has adequate storage and handling capabilities to maintain purchased items in a manner that prevents damage or deterioration. The laboratory shall store received reagents and consumables according to the manufacturer's specifications.

REMARKS

The laboratory has ultimate responsibility for all the results that it generates. While you are responsible to do what you can throughout the life of a reagent, when you take a reagent or consumable into inventory, the responsibility shifts directly to you. There are many ways of managing this duty, but we recommend you: a) document the dates reagents are received; b) record the temperature of the materials on delivery; c) perform acceptance testing on new lots and shipments of reagents; d) segregate or quarantine untested and unacceptable reagents from those in use; e) document the dates reagents go into service (are opened); and f) document any changes in expiration date from opening or manipulating reagents.

We also recommend you employ a first in/first out reagent management system. This will help with both lot control and minimizing reagent expiry and waste. This system will also help save your lab time and money.

The laboratory is also responsible for assuring temperature within storage areas are monitored and appropriate for all reagents stored. This monitoring must ensure proper storage seven days a week (possible with min/max thermometers). This includes refrigerators, freezers, and room temperature. You also need a procedure to describe your corrective actions if you find temperatures out-of-range. This doesn't mean you need to discard all reagents when storage temperatures are exceeded. Rather, the lab must have a procedure to check that reagents stored at improper temperatures for a short period of time are still performing properly.

5.3.2.3 Reagents and Consumables – Acceptance Testing

Each new formulation of examination kits with changes in reagents or procedure, or a new lot or shipment, shall be verified for performance before use in examinations.

Consumables that can affect the quality of examination shall be verified for performance before use in examinations.

REMARKS

It is a long journey for reagents and consumables to be delivered from the manufacturer to your laboratory and much can go wrong. As such, QMS-compliant laboratories cannot assume these reagents and consumables are acceptable for testing until it is confirmed they are. After assuring the environmental conditions during transit were up to standard by measuring the temperature, the next step is moving the reagents and consumables into inventory and wait until they are placed into service. The laboratory must also ensure that these untested reagents and consumables are not accidentally used (see 5.3.2.4). Before using them, the laboratory must confirm that the reagents and relevant consumables are still within specification. The most practical way to do so is to simply run controls and known patient samples using the old lot of reagents you are about to replace alongside the new lot.

Remember when we refer to lots, we are discussing two things. One is the manufacturer's lot based on production. The other is the lot of reagents or supplies that were inventoried into your lab. Often, new production lots and shipping lots are one and the same, but not always. If you fail to run correlations in both cases, some nasty quality surprises may await. To be in compliance with ISO 15189, you must test all new lots and all new shipments of the same lot.

5.3.2.4 Reagents and Consumables – Inventory Management

The laboratory shall establish an inventory control system for reagents and consumables. The system for inventory control shall segregate uninspected and unacceptable reagents and consumables from those that have been accepted for use.

REMARKS

The lab is a busy place. If you store together as-yet non-validated reagents and consumables (or even worse, those with a proven record of incompatibility) with your primary supply, someone will inevitably make a mistake and grab the wrong material. At best this mistake will cost your laboratory time and money. At worst, you may report erroneous results and harm patients.

There are many ways of ensuring non-verified or problem reagents/supplies are not used by mistake. Separation and clear labeling are the simplest ways. If you have to inventory large volumes of reagents for high-volume testing, labeled trays and a first in/first out inventory system can work well provided you use easy-to-read tabs that clearly identify lot changes and verified versus non-verified status.

For problem reagents, you may want to avoid disposal either for refund purposes or to show the manufacturer as a form of QC. If you do keep these kinds of problematic reagents, we suggest labeling them with a big red "X" and "DEFECTIVE! DO NOT USE!". Be sure to contact your vendor as well. There may be a problem either with the whole lot or just with your shipment, and they may be required to refund your account or provide new reagents free-of-charge. This provision is important to put in your contract with the vendor.

5.3.2.5 Reagents and Consumables - Instructions for Use

Instructions for use of reagents and consumables, including those provided by the manufacturers, shall be readily available.

REMARKS

Most reagents come with package inserts applicable to each set of products. One simple technique is to take the insert and file it or display it near the actual testing site/bench/location. More difficult, however, is ensuring that those doing the testing have actually read or understood the insert contents. Adding to this complexity, package inserts can change over time. Confirming that your people have read and understood the content of package inserts should be included as part of the competency assessment you are required to carry out (refer to FOS Competency Assessment and Performance Review in the Personnel Department).

Managing the complexities of package insert changes is a different thing altogether. To simply things for their customers, many reagent manufacturers mark their boxes whenever a significant change has been made to the package insert. If the product is manufactured by a US company and regulated by the FDA, this kind of insert signposting is mandatory.

When dealing with unregulated assays with no manufacturer notifications, the only way to know if there has been a significant change is to review the new and old package inserts side-by-side. Naturally, this is a horribly tedious process, but the negative consequences of these significant changes (be it software settings, assay protocols, or units) constitute major risk factors. In fact, it might be a good idea to add "Prominent Notification of Package Insert Changes" to your instrument and reagent pre-acquisition checklist.

5.3.2.7 Reagents and Consumables – Records

Records shall be maintained for each reagent and consumable that contributes to the performance of examinations.

The records shall include, but not limited to, the following:

a) Identity of the reagent or consumable;
b) Manufacturer's name and batch code or lot number;
c) Contact information for the supplier or manufacturer;
d) Date of receiving, the expiry date, date of entering into service and, where applicable, the date the material was taken out of service;
e) Condition when received (e.g., acceptable or damaged) ;
f) Manufacturer's instructions;
g) Records that confirm the reagent's or consumable's initial acceptance for use;
h) Performance records that confirm the reagent's or consumable's ongoing acceptance for use.

Where the laboratory uses reagents prepared or completed in-house, the records shall include, in addition to the relevant information above, reference to the person or persons undertaking their preparation and the date of preparation.

REMARKS

Maintaining accurate and complete records of your reagents and consumables will pay great dividends when troubleshooting quality control, instrument performance, and people problems. Of course, you can create a separate and independent log containing all of this information but a more practical approach for maintaining these records is to assimilate this information into other areas of your QMS documentation. Refer to the templates included in this FOS to determine which method works best for your laboratory.

Why being in compliance with this FOS is important:

Things that can go wrong if your reagents or consumables are compromised are too long to list. These include poor results potentially leading to compromised patient outcomes, spending staff time trying to troubleshoot problems, and lower productivity. It can also lead to expensive repeat testing and poor turnaround times.

On the other hand, the effort of properly managing your reagents and consumables can pay great dividends. If done properly, problems can be found quickly, and responsible partners can be made accountable. This is especially true when making claims to manufacturers backed with the proper documentation about reagents coming in with short expiration dating or out-of-temperature specifications. You will be able to track the number of tests reported versus the number of tests run, potentially plugging expensive processes or quality control errors.

Materials Included In This FOS
• Reagents and Consumables Management Policies and Procedures
• Reagents and Consumables Log
• Contact List of Manufacturers
• Reagent Label Form
• Lot-to-Lot Comparison Data
• Package Inserts for Reagents and Consumables
• Prominent Notification of Package Insert Changes

FOS: Instrument & Equipment Selection, Acquisition & Acceptance / ISO 5.3, 5.3.1, 5.3.1.1, 5.3.1.2

5.3 Laboratory Equipment, Reagents and Consumables

NOTE 1: For the purpose of this International Standard, laboratory equipment includes hardware and software of instruments, measuring systems, and laboratory information systems.

NOTE 2: Reagents include reference materials, calibrators and quality control materials; consumables include culture media, pipette tips, glass slides, etc.

NOTE 3: See 4.6 for information concerning the selection and purchasing of external services, equipment, reagents and consumables.

5.3.1 Equipment

5.3.1.1 General

The laboratory shall have a documented procedure for the selection, purchasing and management of equipment.

The laboratory shall be furnished with all equipment needed for the provision of services (including primary sample collection, sample preparation, sample processing, examination and storage).

In cases where the laboratory needs to use equipment outside its permanent control, laboratory management shall ensure that the requirements of this International Standard are met.

The laboratory shall replace equipment as needed to ensure the quality of examination results.

REMARKS

The equipment selection process begins with an analysis of your users' testing needs. The best way to start is by creating a sheet with several columns consisting of:

a) Test name
b) Current testing volume
c) Anticipated testing volume

Once you understand user needs, the next step is researching suitable and available instruments, methodologies, and/or equipment. If this information is not available on the Internet, a local sales rep surely can help you. You may also find your own employees experienced on a variety of equipment platforms. Your Gap Analysis should include the following three critical elements: 1) performance; 2) support; and 3) economics. For each element, ask the following questions.

Performance

a) Does the equipment meet your current testing throughput requirements?
b) Does the equipment meet your future testing throughput requirements?
c) What is the mean time between failures?
d) What is the precision and accuracy within clinical requirements?
e) How does the assay perform on third-party external surveys?
f) Interface-ability with current or future LIS?
g) Will normal ranges match those of your current system?
h) What is the dynamic range of each assay?
i) What is the published sensitivity and specificity?
j) Will the equipment function within your laboratory environment (temperature, humidity, etc.)?
k) Are the specimen stability requirements (time and temperature) achievable in your system?
l) Is the proficiency testing peer group of sufficient size for meaningful intra-laboratory comparisons?
m) Does the instrument prevent reporting results when QC is out-of-range?
n) Does the instrument lock you out if reagents are expired?

Support

a) How long has the system been on the market and how long will the manufacturer support it?
b) What service guarantees are available?
c) Training availability?
d) Manufacturer's recall track record?
e) Forecasted upgrades to testing menu and/or functionality?
f) Available support for correlation and assay validation?
g) Internet connectivity for performance monitoring?
h) Availability of supplies?
i) Can you interface the equipment to your LIS? Is the interface bidirectional?
j) Are there sufficient checks to support autoverification (if volume dictates)?

Economics

a) What is the expected life of the equipment?
b) Amortized cost of the equipment based on the life expectancy?
c) Projected cost for supplies?
d) Cost of an annual service contract?
e) Training costs?
f) What is the cost of validation and correlation?
g) What is the fully burdened cost per-result when calculating all the above factors?
h) How much will the vendor and LIS-vendor charge for an LIS interface?
i) How easy is it to scale if your volume increases?
j) How long are you locked into a contract if volume decreases?
k) Are the reagent shelf lives and lot runs sufficient to keep lot-to-lot testing cost low?
l) What are the storage requirements of reagents (temperature and size)?

After assembling your date, you must then critically analyze all these factors and base your decision on the lab's best interests. Since the optimum decisions tend to be a combination of factors, you cannot merely choose, say, the best performance or best service support or the cheapest. Ultimately, the system you choose will only meet your needs if it satisfies your lab's workflow requirements and those of your clients.

5.3.1.2 Equipment Acceptance Testing

The laboratory shall verify upon installation and before use that the equipment is capable of achieving the necessary performance and that it complies with the requirements relevant to any examinations concerned (see also 5.5.1).

NOTE: This requirement applies to equipment used in the laboratory, equipment on loan or equipment used in associated or mobile facilities by others authorized by the laboratory.

Each item of equipment shall be uniquely labeled, marked or otherwise identified.

REMARKS

Given the quality of modern instrumentation and equipment, it is easy to trust the manufacturers and feel confident that the equipment you carefully selected and purchased (based on strict criteria) lives up to its anticipated specifications. Even if this is the case, you need to remember one thing above all else: it is NOT the manufacturer's responsibility to ensure quality patient care—it is YOURS! Before you press any new equipment into full service, you must first do due diligence. Of course your lab's policies concerning new equipment will dictate to some degree how this happens, but, at the same time, you should keep some of the following examples in mind.

For measuring devices such as pipettes and scales:

- Confirm accuracy

For temperature-dependent devices like water baths, refrigerators, and freezers:

- Confirm actual vs. published temperatures

For speed-dependent devices like centrifuges:

- Confirm actual vs. published RPM

For computers, software, and LIS:

- Check everything, especially reporting units, decimal placement, and data transmission accuracy

For analytical instrumentation:

- Check correlation of results between prior and current instrumentation
- Confirm actual vs. published analytical measurement range (AMR)/dynamic range
- Confirm normal ranges
- Confirm interfering substances
- Confirm no carryover
- Confirm linearity, accuracy, and precision
- Confirm low-end sensitivity
- Confirm calibrations

Why being in compliance with this FOS is important:

Choosing the best instrumentation for your laboratory and making sure the instrumentation is operating properly prior to placing it into service can assure you provide the proper level of service to your users. You also avoid many possible risks such as excess instrumentation (costing extra money) or something inadequate that doesn't meet your needs.

The process also helps ensure that there is continuity in testing results so that users are informed in the case of shifts in normal range. It also helps assure against long-term aberrant result reporting.

Compliance to these standards will help your lab both economically and help fulfill your mission for facilitating quality patient outcomes.

Materials Included In This FOS
• Instrument and Equipment Selection, Acquisition and Acceptance Policies and Procedures
• Acquisition Request, Acceptance and Implementation Form

FOS: Instrument & Equipment Instructions, Calibration & Maintenance / ISO 5.3.1.3, 5.3.1.4, 5.3.1.5, 5.3.1.7

5.3.1.3 Equipment Instructions for Use

Equipment shall be operated at all times by trained and authorized personnel.

Current instructions on the use, safety and maintenance of equipment, including any relevant manuals and directions for use provided by the manufacturer of the equipment, shall be readily available.

The laboratory shall have procedures for safe handling, transport, storage and use of equipment to prevent its contamination or deterioration.

REMARKS

Training on major analytical systems is usually available from manufacturers. If training takes place in the lab, however, we highly recommend that trainees be given a very focused experience that stresses learning and retention. In a busy workplace, this can be challenging; therefore, when possible, we believe off-site training is always preferable. If off-site training cannot be provided, ensure the trainees have sufficient time away from their other clinical duties to complete their training uninterrupted.

If your trainee is, or will be, a primary operator, we encourage you to choose someone who is not only qualified and a solid learner but also a person who can effectively communicate what they have learned to others and later train their colleagues, as required. Also, make sure you instruct your main trainees to request copies of all presentations and other training materials so you can use these later for your own internal training.

Finally, do not forget to have someone maintain these files/materials as they will be useful later for cross-training of existing, new, or transferred staff.

If standardized training is not available, we suggest you evaluate the new system package inserts and create courses based on that information or in combination with increasingly available online courses.

Regardless of the training type or style, make sure it is documented in either the personnel files or training logs, or, in some cases, both.

5.3.1.4 Equipment Calibration and Metrological Traceability

The laboratory shall have a documented procedure for the calibration of equipment that directly or indirectly affects examination results. This procedure includes:

a) Taking into account conditions of use and the manufacturer's instructions;
b) Recording the metrological traceability of the calibration standard and the traceable calibration of the item of equipment;
c) Verifying the required measurement accuracy and the functioning of the measuring system at defined intervals;
d) Recording the calibration status and date of recalibration;
e) Ensuring that, where calibration gives rise to a set of correction factors, the previous calibration factors are correctly updated;
f) Safeguards to prevent adjustments or tampering that might invalidate examination results.

Metrological traceability shall be a reference material or reference procedure of the higher metrological order available.

NOTE: Documentation of calibration traceability to a higher reference material or reference procedure may be provided by an examination system manufacturer. Such documentation is acceptable as long as the manufacturer's examination system and calibration procedures are used without modification. Where it is not possible or relevant, other means for providing confidence in the results shall be applied, including but not limited to the following:

- Use of certified reference material;
- Examination or calibration by another procedure;

- Mutual consent standards or methods which are clearly established, specified, characterized and mutually agreed upon by all parties concerned.

REMARKS

For nearly all calibration procedures, there are generally two major variables we want to eliminate:

1) The reproducible technique and skill of the person performing the calibration
2) The accuracy of the reference materials

When we refer to "traceability," we are talking about confirming and documenting the reliability of reference materials. The question to ask is: can you trace the accuracy of each piece of equipment to a trustworthy, documented source which is compliant with ISO standards?

When we use manufacturer-provided materials, we trust that the manufacturer only employs certified, standard materials. If your lab is not using manufacturer-produced materials, however, it is important that you check the accuracy of the source materials and document sources yourself.

If you calibrated an assay using an inaccurate source material or measure with an inaccurate measurement method, for example, you would not only be yielding inaccurate results but could also be doing so long-term without even knowing it. Here are some troubling scenarios:

a) You regularly check the water bath you employ with ELISA testing. The method calls for the water to be 37 degrees Celsius +/– 0.5 degrees. You have not confirmed the accuracy of this thermometer, however, and it is actually reading 1.2 degrees lower than standard. RESULT: All ELISA calibrations, controls, and patient results are reported lower than manufacturer specifications.
b) You use a pipette for measuring a pre-treatment for a neonatal assay. The pipette is new and assumed accurate. In actuality, the 5 uL is actually pipetting 6.2 uL. RESULT: All assays are reported high.

c) You are storing reagents in a refrigerator and dutifully recording the temperature daily using an electronic thermometer you bought at a supermarket. You assumed it was accurate enough. The manufacturer storage requirements call for 2-8 degrees Celsius. The thermometer is reading 3 degrees lower than the actual temperature. RESULT: 40% of the documented temperature readings are out-of-range. Many of your reagents may have deteriorated, causing inaccurate reporting.

In all these situations, there is a single common denominator: the instrumentation used was not calibrated to a certified equivalent or reference standard. If someone is going to use uncertified material or measuring device, they need to ascertain accuracy against a certified source and document this source prior to placing it into service. We further recommend this be done periodically. In our opinion, all devices need to be re-certified against a reliable standard even after seemingly small incidents like a drop or an earthquake.

We highly recommend that the calibration of ancillary equipment be performed by an ISO 17025-accredited laboratory. *NOTE: This does not apply to manufacturer-calibrated equipment that is FDA or other governmental body-approved.*

If you choose to do calibrations in-house, you must fully comply with these standards. This includes training and competency assessments of performing calibrations, adequate documentation of methods and labeling of accredited equipment, producing compliant calibration certificates, calculating measurement uncertainty of your calibrations. As you can see, this can be very involved for a clinical laboratory and may be best accomplished by outsourcing these calibrations to a qualified lab.

When you outsource your calibrations, ensure that the laboratory you contact with is ISO 17025-accredited, that their scope of testing covers the instruments that you're using, and that the range of their scope covers your calibration ranges. Lastly, be aware that some companies offer several tiers of service, some of which do not include measurement uncertainty and compliance with the ISO 17025 Standard. Ensure that you include these requirements in your contract.

5.3.1.5 Equipment Maintenance and Repair

The laboratory shall have a documented program of preventative maintenance which, at a minimum, follows the manufacturer's instructions.

Equipment shall be maintained in a safe working condition and in working order. This shall include examination of electrical safety, emergency stop devices where they exist, and the safe handling and disposal of chemical, radioactive and biological materials by authorized persons.

At a minimum, manufacturer's schedules or instructions, or both, shall be used.

Whenever equipment is found to be defective, it shall be taken out of service and clearly labeled. The laboratory shall ensure that defective equipment is not used until it has been repaired and shown by verification to meet specified acceptance criteria.

The laboratory shall examine the effect of any defects on previous examinations and institute immediate action or corrective action (see 4.10).

The laboratory shall take reasonable measures to decontaminate equipment before service, repair or decommissioning, provide suitable space for repairs and provide appropriate personnel protective equipment.

When equipment is removed from the direct control of the laboratory, the laboratory shall ensure that its performance is verified before being returned to laboratory use.

REMARKS

In all likelihood, the largest preventable mistakes and problems that occur in clinical labs happen because of little or no routine maintenance. As the saying goes, an ounce of prevention is worth a pound of cure.

Most equipment (including computers and software) and instrumentation come with preventative maintenance instructions. Maintenance may be required on a daily, weekly, monthly, and quarterly basis. Typically, routine maintenance is the lab staff's responsibility.

For larger systems, most manufacturers offer preventative maintenance programs that are typically every six months or yearly. First-year programs typically are included in the instrument warranty. For subsequent years, preventative maintenance is done on a service-contract basis. These service agreement costs may vary and may be front-loaded onto the cost of the instrument in some cases. Lease arrangements are also common. As a general rule, annual service contracts are about 10% of the cost of the analyzer.

Whenever manufacturers provide preventative maintenance (or any service), we recommend you insist they leave a written record of exactly what they did and what they found during the preventative maintenance or service visit. Preventative maintenance can lead to shifts in quality control, especially if major systems such as optics are replaced or manipulated. Some laboratories mandate re-calibration of all assays after major maintenance or repair. Remember, manufacturer representatives are human too and can make mistakes. At the very least, we recommend you run QC after all preventative maintenance or major service calls.

If the manufacturer requires daily maintenance, the schedule must be kept and the maintenance documented (see 5.3.1.7 below). It is also best practice to have a supervisor or lead tech check the performance of the daily or other routine maintenance performed by lab staff at least on a monthly basis. Ensure that the individuals who perform the maintenance and reviews are qualified and that the delegation is in writing.

5.3.1.7 Equipment Records

Records shall be maintained for each item of equipment that contributes to the performance of examinations. The equipment records shall include, but not be limited to, the following:

a) Identity of the equipment;
b) Manufacturer's name, model and serial number or other unique identification;
c) Contact information for the supplier or the manufacturer;
d) Date of receiving and date of entering in service;

e) Location;
f) Condition when received (e.g., new, used or reconditioned);
g) Manufacturer's instructions;
h) Records that confirmed the equipment's initial acceptability for use when equipment is incorporated in the laboratory;
i) Maintenance carried out and the schedule for preventative maintenance;
j) Equipment performance records that confirm the equipment's ongoing acceptability for use;
k) Damage to, or malfunction, modification or repair of the equipment.

The performance records referred to in j) shall include copies of reports/certificates of all calibrations and/or verifications including dates, times and results, adjustments, the acceptance criteria and due date of the next calibration and/or verification, to fulfill part or all of this requirement.

These records shall be maintained and shall be readily available for the lifespan of the equipment or longer, as specified in the laboratory's control of records procedures (see 4.13).

REMARKS

Lab instrumentation and equipment are essential tools. As the reliability of these systems improves, it is easy for us to slowly let our guard down and neglect the maintenance all these tools need to stay at peak performance. You may escape noticeable problems by not performing required maintenance for a short time, but, long-term, this failure will come back to haunt you and your lab in major ways. Ongoing instrument maintenance is critical, and the only way to manage the process is through meticulous documentation.

Why being in compliance with this FOS is important:

If you don't maintain a system, it will become sub- or non-operational. You will induce variability in your results and decrease testing quality. In the case of sub-optimal performance, patient results may be incorrectly reported. In the case of non-operational systems, you will experience delay in both testing and reporting.

You may also shorten the life expectancy of your equipment, and it may very well cost you more money in the long-term. In either case, it will degrade the level of patient care, impact the reputation of your laboratory, and cause your laboratory economic harm. You will also not be certified to maintain ISO 15189 accreditation.

Materials Included In This FOS
• Instrument and Equipment Instructions, Calibrations and Maintenance Policies and Procedures
• Instrument and Equipment Log
• Instructions for Use of Instruments and Equipment
• Instrument and Equipment Maintenance Log
• Established Standard Certifications
• Calibration Log
• Calibration Seal

FOS: Review of Suitability of Procedures & Sample Requirements / ISO 4.14.2

4.14.2 Periodic Review of Requests and Suitability of Procedures and Sample Requirements

Authorized personnel shall periodically review the examinations provided by the laboratory to ensure that they are clinically appropriate for the requests received.

The laboratory shall periodically review its sample volume, collection device and preservative requirements for blood, urine, other body fluids, tissue and other sample types, as applicable, to ensure that neither insufficient nor excessive amounts of samples are collected and the sample is properly collected to preserve the measured.

REMARKS

Note that this FOS is included in the overarching general lab FOS, but the details should be managed at the department level. You should remain aware that the information collected within this FOS can affect a number of FOSs in different departments (e.g., sample collection department, quality assurance department, and technical departments). Any changes in procedures and sample requirements should be accurately and promptly reflected and notified to relevant persons including users, if necessary. Ideally, each technical department should assess the suitability of the procedures and sample requirements based on their expertise, notify the quality assurance department in case any necessary changes are identified, and the relevant documentation (e.g., Laboratory Test Guide, Test Requisition Forms, Assay SOPs, etc.) should be modified accordingly.

As technology advances and new instrumentation and methods are introduced into the market, the laboratory needs to ensure that the instrumentation, methodologies, sample collection methods, etc., are truly adequate to support their users' needs. While client satisfaction and such are generally managed by the quality assurance department, it is the technical department's responsibility to assess the procedures implemented from an expert point-of-view.

Why being in compliance with this FOS is important:

Methodologies are continuously changing with decreases in sample size requirements. Given such progress, the laboratory will need a system that reviews your current methods as well as any new technologies available to determine if changes are required, especially to ensure that your samples are as small as possible. It is worth noting that newer and smaller sample sizes may positively affect patient comfort and clinical implications. What's more, they may even help alleviate storage capacity issues and economic burden.

Materials Included In This FOS
• Review of Suitability of Procedures and Sample Requirements Policies and Procedures
• Procedures and Sample Requirement Review Log
• Request for Change in Laboratory Documentation

FOS: Testing Documentation / ISO 5.5.3

5.5.3 Documentation of Examination Procedures

Examination procedures shall be documented.

They shall be written in a language commonly understood by the staff in the laboratory and be available in appropriate locations.

Any condensed document format (e.g., card files or similarly used systems) shall correspond to the documented procedure.

NOTE 1: Working instructions, card files or similar systems that summarize key information are acceptable for use as a quick reference at the work-bench, provided that a full documented procedure is available for reference.

NOTE 2: Information from product instructions for use may be incorporated into examination procedures by reference.

All documents that are associated with the performance of examinations, including procedures, summary documents, condensed document format and product instructions for use, shall be subject to document control.

In addition to document control identifiers, documentation shall include, when applicable to the examination procedure, the following:

a) Purpose of the examination;
b) Principle and method of the procedure used for examinations;
c) Performance characteristics (see 5.5.1.2 and 5.5.1.3);
d) Type of sample (e.g., plasma, serum, urine);
e) Patient preparation;
f) Type of container and additives;
g) Required equipment and reagents;
h) Environmental and safety controls;
i) Calibration procedures (metrological traceability);
j) Procedural steps;
k) Quality control procedures;

l) Interferences (e.g., lipemia, hemolysis, bilirubinemia, drugs) and cross reactions;
m) Principle of procedure for calculating results including, where relevant, the measurement uncertainty of measured quantity values;
n) Biological reference intervals or clinical decision values;
o) Reportable interval of examination results;
p) Instructions for determining quantitative results when a result is not within the measurement interval;
q) Alert/critical values, where appropriate;
r) Laboratory clinical interpretation ;
s) Potential sources of variation;
t) References.

If the laboratory intends to change existing examination procedure such that results or their interpretations could be significantly different, the implications shall be explained to users of the laboratory services after validating the procedure.

NOTE 3: This requirement can be accomplished in different ways depending on local circumstances. Some methods include directed mailings, laboratory newsletters or part of the examination report itself.

REMARKS

The key points here are:

1) Have complete procedures available for each assay
2) If you use bench notes, make sure they remain consistent with the main procedure and are controlled
3) Use a well-managed document control system to ensure procedures remain up-to-date so you can easily identify the most current procedure
4) If you make changes potentially impacting patients, ensure clients get informed
5) Ensure that procedures are readily available to the individuals performing the testing
6) Ensure that your employees (including pathologists) are familiar with appropriate procedures

Why being in compliance with this FOS is important:

Not correctly documenting processes for each analyte tested may result in incorrect use and corresponding incorrect results or interpretation of results. When changes in an analyte SOP are not reflected in the bench notes or if the document management system leaves old versions of an SOP near the laboratory bench, these are common errors in assay processing and interpretation and can lead to medical errors. These problems have been known to persist for long periods and impact large numbers of patients.

Materials Included In This FOS
• Testing Documentation Policies and Procedures
• SOPs for Each Assay
• Source Information for Assay SOPs

FOS: Quality Control / ISO 5.6, 5.6.1, 5.6.2, 5.6.2.1, 5.6.2.2, 5.6.2.3

5.6 Ensuring Quality of Examination Results

5.6.1 General

The laboratory shall ensure the quality of examinations by performing them under defined conditions.

Appropriate pre- and post-examination processes shall be implemented (see 4.14.7, 5.4, 5.7 and 5.8).

The laboratory shall not fabricate any results.

REMARKS

Most trained lab technicians will be familiar with quality control (QC). Having said that, let's examine the concept of "fabricating results" mentioned in 5.6.1 above. As we all know and surely agree, constructing false patient test results is one of the most horrendous acts a laboratory can commit. *BUT, it does happen.* There are hundreds of cases of "sink testing" reported annually in the United States alone. As you can imagine, the consequences are devastating for patient care (and for the offending technologists as well as they may face criminal action if discovered—possibly even as accessory to murder).

Monitoring for sink testing on larger scales can be done simply enough; just calculate average reagent usage by the number of tests reported and investigate any abnormalities.

Fabricating quality control results is also harmful. Of course, everyone wants to be proud of his/her QC results, but false reporting hurts everyone. One small example of how this might happen is a result that falls out of range; the test then gets re-run with a proper range but with the original poor result going unrecorded. This would constitute a fabricated result. If perfect QC results are due to the re-running of controls until one comes into range and not recording the out-of-range results, that is *not* QC.

Finally, everyone must understand that fabricating QC results can be even more damaging than sink testing single patient samples. It destroys the integrity of the process and can thus affect large numbers of patient results.

5.6.2 Quality Control

5.6.2.1 General

The laboratory shall design quality control procedures that verify the attainment of the intended quality of results.

NOTE: In several countries, quality control, as referred to in this subclause, is also named "internal quality control".

REMARKS

There are vast resources available that discuss internal quality control; therefore, we will not labor the point except briefly to bring up "clinical relevancy". The truth is we can become obsessed with refining quality control—and why not? It is at the core of what we do, and we should take pride in doing the best we can. If so, we cannot ignore the concept of "diminishing returns". For example, if you have an assay running with two standard deviations and you have evaluated this to satisfy the precision necessary for clinical interpretation, is there any value in expending resources to drive the standard deviation to 1.0? Beyond academic curiosity, the answer is probably no. As with all things under ISO, the degree of precision needed is dictated by the needs of the user. In the case of medical testing, this is largely driven by clinical utility.

This brings us to another point: blanket quality control rules. Some labs, for example, arbitrarily determine Coefficient of Variation (CV) and Standard Deviation (SD), and these are made applicable across all testing methods. Instead, we recommend you evaluate each testing method and then answer the question: what is the clinical tolerance? In some cases, a CV of 3.0 could be fine. In other situations, you will need to work hard to improve your QC so you can satisfy your user and clinical relevancy requirements.

Quality control has several defined rule sets. Perhaps the most widely used are the Westgard Rules, which are a set of rules that can be applied separately to each test based on clinical risk and other factors. We encourage your lab to examine the Westgard Rules and see if implementing them for particular tests is appropriate. If you are a CAP-accredited laboratory, you will need to institute IQCP rules for each test that is undergoing QC at a frequency less than what CAP or CLIA allows. This is required even if that lower frequency for QC is permitted by the test manufacturer. Under IQCP, you must establish QC frequency for each assay based on risk factors.

Lastly, there are a multitude of software products to help you record, analyze, and report quality control results as well as with auto-verification programs. While these can all be outstanding tools, they are only as good as the data reviewing process and how the lab staff use it.

5.6.2.2 Quality Control Materials

The laboratory shall use quality control materials that react to the examining system in a manner as close as possible to patient samples.

Quality control materials shall be periodically examined with a frequency that is based on the stability of the procedure and the risk of harm to the patient from an erroneous result.

NOTE 1: The laboratory should choose concentrations of control materials, wherever possible, especially at or near clinical decision values, which ensure the validity of decisions made.

NOTE 2: Use of independent third party control materials should be considered, either instead of or in addition to any control materials supplied by the reagent or instrument manufacturer.

REMARKS

There are several ways to source quality control materials. These include: a) controls purchased through a test vendor, either as part of a kit or separately; b) third party commercial controls; and c) validated pooled specimens.

Increasingly, the most common controls used in many countries are those included in commercial kits. These controls are often optimized for the particular kit, so you tend not to get any surprises. But many feel, like an audit with no findings, that optimized, vendor supplied controls do not really test the system. They feel that third party controls are more academically honest and reveal problems that would not come to light with manufacturer's control material.

Using pooled specimens can be seen as an economic option for controls because your cost of the control material is essentially free in the form of excess patient samples. But these seemingly economic options can be deceiving when you look at the time and effort required to validate and verify these controls. Especially problematic can be attempts at providing control values covering the entire reportable range. It is for these reasons that, in many places, pooled controls are falling out of favor versus commercially available systems that come pre-validated and cover an appropriate spectrum of results.

There is something to note on control materials that can be important, especially with third party controls or pooled specimens. Many times, these controls may contain stabilizers and preservatives to extend their useful shelf life. These substances may interfere with some assay systems, such as the matrix effect seen with dry-chemistry. You always need to remember that controls are, by definition, different than patient samples due to added stabilizers, and this needs to be considered when troubleshooting out-of-range control results.

5.6.2.3 Quality Control Data

The laboratory shall have a procedure to prevent the release of patient results in the event of quality control failure.

When the quality control rules are violated and indicate that examination results are likely to contain clinically significant errors, the results shall be rejected and relevant patient samples re-examined after the error condition has been corrected and within-specification performance is verified. The laboratory shall also evaluate the results from patient samples that were examined after the last successful quality control event.

Quality control data shall be reviewed at regular intervals to detect trends in examination performance that may indicate problems in the examination system. When such trends are noted, preventative actions shall be taken and recorded.

NOTE: Statistical and non-statistical techniques for process control should be used wherever possible to continuously monitor examination system performance.

REMARKS

A complete discussion of evaluating quality control results is beyond the scope of this book. However, there are some important things to keep in mind. First, you need to establish acceptable QC ranges based on risk. Second, you need to evaluate control data before reporting results. And, lastly, if you are using an auto-verification system, it is essential to test this system regularly to ensure that results are not reported with out-of-range controls. The best way to do this is to purposely include control materials you know will be out-of-range and determine if your auto-verification system flags this prior to reporting results.

Why being in compliance with this FOS is important:

Falsifying results could kill people, land the fabricator in jail, and cause civil and criminal penalties for the laboratory and its director. Quality control materials that only evaluate a part of the reportable range will leave many results essentially non-controlled. Using inappropriate control materials will cause you to repeat results and spend a great deal of time troubleshooting. And lastly, not evaluating results properly is tantamount to not doing quality control at all. All of these things can lead to baked-in errors that can impact the care of thousands of patients.

Materials Included In This FOS
• Quality Control Policies and Procedures
• Quality Control SOP

FOS: Risk Management / ISO 4.14.6

4.14.6 Risk Management

The laboratory shall evaluate the impact of work processes and potential failures on examination results as they affect patient safety, and shall modify processes to reduce or eliminate the identified risks and document decisions and actions taken.

REMARKS

Within the world of ISO, the definition of risk is a random event that has a negative impact (as defined in ISO 15190). There are two components to risk: the probability of occurrence of harm and the severity of that harm. Laboratory risk management involves the assessment of both these components of risk and applying the risk assessment into prioritization of QMS activities and into performance of these activities.

There are a number of tools available to help with risk assessment and management; process mapping, fishbone diagrams, and risk grading systems. Our advice is to keep things simple. Use tools that are most helpful or that you are most familiar with to analyze risk. Risk management is best as a team where you have the diversity of inputs and opinions to address issues and find solutions.

To comply with this standard, first and foremost, you need to be vigilant. Look for problems everywhere at all times. To be effective, this vigilance needs to be instilled in everyone at all levels of the laboratory. As 4.14.6 largely depends on Nonconformities (4.9, 4.10, 4.11) and Quality Indicators (4.14.7), these FOSs are included in each technical department as well.

There are two kinds of risk that require management. First are problems that are already "symptomatic," that is, the results of the problem are already causing harm, and these should be dealt with immediately. Note that the objective of having a Risk Management Program is to identify and adopt measure that will either solve or prevent risks prior to them becoming "symptomatic" (i.e., before harm is caused).

Issues that can potentially impact patient safety are numerous and occur at all levels. Examples of risks for each stage include:

Pre-examination

a. Failure by the clinician to collect a proper sample
b. Failure associated to samples adhering to environmental or maximum time-to-assay standards
c. Excessive lipemia, hemolysis, or icteric samples
d. Malfunctions of refrigerators containing patient samples prior to assays being performed
e. Failure to collect patient demographic information such as age, gender, and clinical conditions which help identify samples and may be relevant to test results

Examination

a. Failure to review quality control prior to release of results and discovering post-fact that the results were not within range
b. Notification by reagent manufacturers concerning a recalled reagent lot you have already reported results from
c. Discovery of a carry-over problem in your system
d. Use of glassware with excess detergent residue
e. Problem employee reporting results without actually performing the tests

Post-examination

a. Transcription error(s) on patient reports
b. Wrong interpretation of test data/results by clinicians
c. Reporting results outside established turnaround time guidelines
d. Mistaking unit of measure noted on patient reports
e. Failure to include age and/or gender in patient reportable assays impacted by these factors

In all cases, the quality assurance department and laboratory director must be notified immediately so that the situation can be dealt with transparently and quickly. The primary objective is *not* to save face with the client. Instead, the goal is to focus solely on the patient: how best to mitigate the problem and decrease morbidity/mortality that might have resulted from such errors.

Identifying a problem and fixing it is typically how these issues get handled. The objective of 4.14.6 is to get the laboratory to proactively identify such risk factors prior to it becoming symptomatic and implement preventative measures and not only corrective measures. Periodic, system-wide analysis of your processes is one way of mitigating and managing risk. We strongly recommend that you include the entire staff in this process and encourage and reward staff members who identify possible risk factors and seek proactive solutions. When these issues are identified, they need to become agenda items for quality meetings so that they can be considered potential quality objectives and/or indicators.

Note that risk management reviews can be combined with internal audits or performed separately. Obviously, an independent review of risk management allows more focus and may be more effective. The results of your risk management activities must also be an input into your management reviews (4.15.2 (e)).

Risk management can involve issues outside of test results and patient safety. There are risks associated with employee safety (e.g., chemical and biological hazards) and legal risks (e.g., storing records for longer than the minimum necessary or longer than required by laboratory policy).

Lastly, risk assessment and management has become a crucial element in determining frequency of QC. The development of an Individual Quality Control Plan (IQCP) may be required when a laboratory departs from daily external QC requirements. These plans include an evaluation of risks associated to not performing daily QC with the level of harm that could result from inaccurate testing to determine the optimum frequency of running quality controls. This may be required, even if your vendor has gotten approval for less frequent quality control. You should refer to your local regulations to see if IQCP is required in your area.

Why being in compliance with this FOS is important:

There are a number of overarching reasons why risk management is important to the laboratory. First, there is the overall moral duty that the laboratory management has to reduce risk to its employees and patients. The implications of not managing risk can have very serious consequences. If unmanaged risks occur, it can seriously weaken the confidence that other areas of the hospital or the public has in the laboratory.

Also, problems in the laboratory tend to be repetitive rather than one-off occurrences. In other words, laboratory problems have a tendency to be baked in and affect many patients over long periods of time. There are noteworthy examples of laboratories reporting out hundreds of thousands or even millions of erroneous results over periods lasting decades. This is why laboratories frequently require a QMS system separate from other hospital departments, and we all need to be on the lookout for these kinds of errors and actively seek to find and fix them.

Risk management not only solves existing problems, but, in its purest state, allows the laboratory to prioritize quality activities and concentrate on tackling issues that pose the greatest risk and fix them before they start.

Materials Included In This FOS
• Risk Management Policies and Procedures
• Individual Quality Control Plan (IQCP)

FOS: Quality Indicators / ISO 4.14.7

4.14.7 Quality Indicators

The laboratory shall establish quality indicators to monitor and evaluate performance throughout critical aspects of pre-examination, examination and post-examination processes.

EXAMPLE: Number of unacceptable samples, number of errors at registration and/or accession, number of corrected reports.

The process of monitoring quality indicators shall be planned, which includes establishing the objectives, methodology, interpretation, limits, action plan and duration of measurement.

The indicators shall be periodically reviewed, to ensure their continued appropriateness.

NOTE 1: Quality indicators to monitor non-examination procedures, such as laboratory safety and environment, completeness of equipment and personnel records, and effectiveness of the document control system may provide valuable management insights.

NOTE 2: The laboratory should establish quality indicators for systematically monitoring and evaluating the laboratory's contribution to patient care (see 4.12).

The laboratory, in consultation with the users, shall establish turnaround times for each of its examinations that reflect clinical needs. The laboratory shall periodically evaluate whether or not it is meeting the established turnaround times.

REMARKS

It's useful to think of creating and maintaining Quality Management Systems (QMS) as a cascade of events. First, you have a quality policy to provide overall guidance. The next step is to provide quality objectives describing specific areas of desired improvement. This stage is followed by one in which you create specific, quantifiable quality indicators to drive your objectives forward.

Your quality objectives and quality indicators are determined by evaluating these objectives and indicators both in terms of fixing problems and also in terms of improvement. Lastly, you must develop target values or performance thresholds for all of your quality indicators. Improvement can occur in several forms such as increases in productivity, safety, economic and—most of all—elevating how the laboratory's work can improve patient outcomes.

Once identified and set-up, these improvement projects need to be tracked and documented until deemed concluded. Concluded objectives and indicators should be replaced by new ones. In the beginning, the laboratory should aim to set up easily achievable objectives and indicators so that staff can grasp the concepts. The number and complexity of these indicators can then be increased over time as understanding improves.

Why being in compliance with this FOS is important:

Areas of desired improvement and the decreasing of risks can only be actionable with a plan and actions. Not executing a quality indicator program will lead to not fixing known problems and not improving upon known areas. This will lead directly to errors and accidents. Executing an effective quality indicator program will drive specific actions that will decrease error, increase productivity, safety and patient outcomes. This is perhaps the most important aspect of your quality journey.

Materials Included In This FOS
• Quality Indicators Policies and Procedures
• Quality Indicators Worksheet

FOS: Evaluation & Audits / ISO 4.14, 4.14.1, 4.14.5, 4.14.8

4.14 Evaluation and Audits

4.14.1 General

The laboratory shall plan and implement the evaluation and internal audit processes needed to:

a) Demonstrate the pre-examination, examination, and post-examination and supporting processes are being conducted in a manner that meets the needs and requirements of users
b) Ensure conformity to the quality management system
c) Continually improve the effectiveness of the quality management system
d) The results of evaluation and improvement activities shall be included in the input to the management review (see 4.15)

NOTE: For improvement activities, see 4.10, 4.11 and 4.12.

4.14.5 Internal Audit

The laboratory shall conduct internal audits at planned intervals to determine whether all activities in the quality management system, including pre-examination, examination, and post-examination:

a) Conform to requirements of this International Standard and to requirements established by the laboratory, and
b) Are implemented, effective, and maintained

NOTE 1: The cycle for internal auditing should normally be completed in one year. It is not necessary that internal audits cover each year, in depth, all elements of the quality management system. The laboratory may decide to focus on a particular activity without completely neglecting the others.

Audits shall be conducted by personnel trained to assess the performance of managerial and technical processes of the quality management system.

The audit program shall take into account the status and importance of the processes and technical and management areas to be audited, as well as the results of previous audits. The audit criteria, scope, frequency, and methods shall be defined and documented.

NOTE 2: See ISO 19011 for guidance.

The laboratory shall have a documented procedure to define the responsibilities and requirements for planning and conducting audits, and for reporting results and maintaining records (see 4.13).

Personnel responsible for the area being audited shall ensure that appropriate action is promptly undertaken when nonconformities are identified. Corrective action shall be taken without undue delay to eliminate the causes of the detected nonconformities (see 4.10).

REMARKS

If you lack special training, we highly recommend working with a trained professional or organization to set up and run your internal auditing processes. This will typically include creating a checklist. We also recommend that you work with someone experienced for your first few internal audits. An effective internal audit is not just about "ticking boxes". Rather, it is about understanding how your underlying systems are functioning day to day.

There are different philosophies about scheduled versus unscheduled audits. Although it is your decision as to how to proceed, as a general rule, the first few audits probably should be scheduled. A schedule gives your staff time to review and address systems prior to the internal audit—which can be very positive in the early days of your QMS journey. In time, however, you may want to consider unscheduled internal audits because in order to obtain real value from your QMS systems, you will need to remain in continuous compliance, 24/7. If your lab is in compliance only in preparation and during an internal or external audit period, you accrue all the cost and work of creating and managing a QMS program with few of the benefits. An audit should reflect your actual day-to-day process and not an artificial state.

LEAP is designed to help you gain and maintain continuous compliance in your QMS 24/7. If you use LEAP as directed, you will be able to detect a breach in your system as soon as it occurs since the QMS Dashboard will notify you when you are out of compliance. LEAP will allow you to identify the department in which the discrepancy occurred, what the discrepancy is (through the department-specific QMS Dashboard), and where corrective measures should be instituted.

Just like complaints or reporting nonconformities, audit findings help the lab to improve processes, procedures, and quality. An audit that repeatedly finds no gap may make the department feel good, but it is largely a waste of effort and has not improved your laboratory's quality.

For bad audits, an immediate search for a scapegoat is likewise not very useful. It is more often than not a process or system issue rather than the fault of an individual. It is best to work together to find a solution.

Lastly, auditors must be trained to perform audits, and objectivity and impartiality must be part of the audit process. Audits also should be independent of the area being audited. This is best done by someone from an independent quality team or someone working in a department different from the one being audited.

4.14.8 Reviews by External Organizations

When reviews by external organizations indicate the laboratory has nonconformities or potential nonconformities, the laboratory shall take appropriate immediate actions and, as warranted, corrective action or preventative action to ensure continuing compliance with the requirements of this International Standard. Records shall be kept of the reviews and of the corrective actions and preventative actions taken.

NOTE: Examples of reviews by external accreditation organizations include: onsite user evaluations, accreditation assessments, regulatory agencies' inspections, and health and safety inspections.

REMARKS

Please refer to the remarks in 4.14.5 about internal audits as all these comments apply equally to external audits.

External audits should be seen as an opportunity for fresh eyes to review your QMS processes. This way, you can confirm your system is working, as well as gain new perspectives and insights. Remember, your auditors visit many labs and see a wide variety of methods—both good and bad—so their knowledge base is broad. Finally, don't forget to ask probing questions and try to get as much as possible out of the investment you are making in the audit process.

It is also helpful if your staff can perform audits of external laboratories. This can be done by participating in accrediting agency peer audits or through informal agreements within or between laboratories. This can be a valuable way to bring some new ideas and processes to your own laboratory. Try to take advantage of all such opportunities.

A fully functioning LEAP can also greatly help you maximize the effectiveness of your external audit. If you correctly populate each of your evidence folders, most of the documented evidence will be available for examination by your external auditor within LEAP. You may also want to consider giving the external auditor access to LEAP during—and perhaps even prior to—the audit. This will give them the opportunity to review all your documentation (if they understand the same language), maximizing the time they spend interacting with your staff. We stress again that an external audit gives you and your staff a prime chance to work with and learn from experts of vast experience and knowledge. Note that you can activate an "inspector" role in LEAP for this purpose. The inspector will have access to all the information stored within LEAP, but they will not have the permission to change any content.

It is only human nature to seek a "good score" on an external audit or any kind of test. However, a perfect result has little value and probably represents a superficial review. Each opportunity for improvement should be seen as helpful. Remember, unless there is an immediate threat to patient or staff safety, you will be given the opportunity to take corrective actions by an external auditor. Do not, however, take this as a license to be unprepared for an external audit—experienced auditors can smell an unprepared lab a mile away. Also, an auditor has limited time and, if overwhelmed by large numbers of easily correctable deficiencies, they may not have time to find all the things that can truly help your laboratory. It is best never to leave anything to chance.

Why being in compliance with this FOS is important:

The internal audit acts as a barometer as to how your laboratory's QMS system is performing. It also allows for open communication, helping to identify points requiring improvement. The external auditing process does the same thing, but from a different, "external" perspective. Internal and external audits act as one of the cornerstones of your QMS, giving you a constant influx of information and supplying your staff meaningful targets for improvement. The results from these audits should be reflected in your quality indicators and help you become a more productive laboratory thereby increasing the lab's contribution to patient outcomes and staff safety.

Materials Included In This FOS
• Evaluation and Audits Policies and Procedures
• Internal Audit Checklist

FOS: Inter-Laboratory Comparisons / ISO 5.6.3, 5.6.3.1, 5.6.3.2, 5.6.3.3, 5.6.3.4

5.6.3 Inter-Laboratory Comparisons

5.6.3.1 Participation

The laboratory shall participate in an inter-laboratory comparison program(s) such as external quality assessment program or proficiency testing program appropriate to the examination and interpretations of examination results. The laboratory shall monitor the results of the inter-laboratory comparison program(s) and participate in the implementation of corrective actions when predetermined performance criteria are not fulfilled.

NOTE: The laboratory should participate in inter-laboratory comparison programs that substantially fulfill the relevant requirements of ISO/IEC 17043.

The laboratory shall establish a documented procedure for inter-laboratory comparison participation that includes defined responsibilities and instructions for participation, and any performance criteria that differ from the criteria used in the inter-laboratory comparison program.

Inter-laboratory comparison program(s) chosen by the laboratory shall, as far as possible, provide clinically relevant challenges that mimic patient samples and have the effect of checking the entire examination process, including pre-examination procedures and post-examination procedures, where possible.

REMARKS

Inter-laboratory comparison programs are also referred to as proficiency testing (PT) programs.

Many professionals consider rigorous PT programs to be one of the most important parts of operating a quality laboratory. Why? Because PT programs represent the chance for one lab to blindly compare all of its internal variables against statistically relevant peer groupings on a per-test methodology basis. To underline the importance of PT, manufacturers and regulatory authorities consistently scour published external PT data to identify possible lapses in their quality systems.

The over 7,000 global College of American Pathologists (CAP)-accredited laboratories, for example, are required to run PT on all tests several times a year. Failure to successfully participate may lead to suspension of a lab's accreditation or requirements to cease some areas of laboratory testing. If CAP PT programs are available in your area, you have no excuse not to participate in external PT for all your tests. Although utilizing CAP PT is not an ISO 15189 requirement, we believe it is one of the best investments you can make.

The best way to negate value from a PT program (and to jeopardize your laboratory's accreditation) is to treat a PT specimen in a manner differently from patient samples (e.g., run it several times, only let certain lab employees perform the testing, and/or perhaps compare results with a manufacturer's rep or friendly lab). Not only would doing this defeat the purpose of using PT, it may mean failing to identify some systemic problem in a manufactured assay system itself.

In some major jurisdictions, cheating on a PT is a crime (fraud). In addition to sanction(s) on the laboratory, loss of accreditation or closure, the individuals and director may also be punished (by the loss of professional licensure, a fine, or even jail).

Most regulatory agencies also have a strict prohibition on communication about PT data or the sharing of PT samples. Ensure your laboratory has a prohibition on such communication until after the deadline for submission of results and that your laboratory notifies appropriate authorities if they ever receive PT samples from another laboratory.

Many manufacturers have inter-laboratory comparison programs available for their customers. These may be appropriate but may also have limitations. These limitations include the fact that, in many cases, samples consist of excess control and calibrator materials that are not representative of normal biological samples. Also, the manufacturers of PT program materials tend to use unnaturally optimized materials that again may not be representative of typical biological specimens and do not challenge potential matrix effects. Some also claim a potential conflict of interest by making them too easy to pass and thus makes manufacturers of PT programs suspect.

Some for-profit manufacturers sell external PT materials. These can be excellent, but purchasers must ensure they don't get a matrix effect from preservatives or other artificial materials. (Some manufacturers use preservatives to promote a longer shelf-life and increased commercial viability.)

We recommend not-for-profit commercial PT suppliers. The world's largest—and arguably the most rigorous—program is administered by CAP. CAP has PT materials for over 1,000 different tests. They also have highly sophisticated analytic procedures that segment results into peer groupings. Over 23,000 clinical laboratories in 72 countries utilize CAP PT programs, and we recommend searching for CAP PT programs available in your area*.

**For purposes of transparency, the producer of LEAP software is also the representative of CAP PT programs in Japan.*

5.6.3.2 Alternative Approaches

Whenever an inter-laboratory comparison is not available, the laboratory shall develop other approaches and provide objective evidence for determining the acceptability of examination results.

Whenever possible, this mechanism shall utilize appropriate materials.

NOTE: Examples of such materials include:

- Certified reference materials;
- Samples previously examined;
- Materials from cell or tissue repositories;
- Exchange of samples with other laboratories;
- Control materials that are tested daily in inter-laboratory comparison programs.

REMARKS

Note that 5.3.2.6 is only applicable if external inter-laboratory comparison programs are *not* available.

There are times when alternative programs are appropriate and necessary, such as when you are using a laboratory-developed assay and externally administered programs are unavailable. Another example would be an assay system that is rare or very new and for which no external programs have been developed. Some distributive test models (such as using bioinformatics analysis at a second lab) are not able to use commercial PT programs because of the prohibition on intra-laboratory comparison. And, if you are one of those unlucky laboratories who still perform bleeding time (and, these days, why are you still doing this test?), it is not a test that allows for external PT. Lastly, some interpretive tests, such as surgical specimens or cytology, are dependent on the competency of those individuals who perform the interpretation. In such instances, a quality peer review program is required to ensure accurate results are reported.

5.6.3.3 Analysis of Inter-Laboratory Comparison Samples

The laboratory shall integrate inter-laboratory comparison samples into the routine workflow in a manner that follows, as much as possible, the handling of patient samples.

Inter-laboratory comparison samples shall be examined by personnel who routinely examine patient samples using the same procedures as those used for samples.

The laboratory shall not communicate with other participants in the inter-laboratory comparison program about sample data until after the date for submission of data.

The laboratory shall not refer inter-laboratory comparison samples for confirmatory examination before submission of the data, although this would routinely be done with patient samples.

5.6.3.4 Evaluation of Laboratory Performance

The performance in inter-laboratory comparisons shall be reviewed and discussed with relevant staff.

When predetermined performance criteria are not fulfilled (i.e., nonconformities are present), staff shall participate in the implementation and recording of corrective action. The effectiveness of corrective action shall be monitored. The returned results shall be evaluated for trends that indicate potential nonconformities and preventative action shall be taken.

REMARKS

The main point here is to stress that *the only time you can be absolutely sure your tests are accurate is at the point of* ***inter-laboratory comparison***. Also, intervals of time between inter-laboratory comparisons need to be considered suspect because they are only being judged by internally regulated systems. This is especially true when any changes of any time occur—and the bigger the change, the bigger the risk. Changes can include relatively routine things like new lots of reagents, calibrators, and control as well as major changes like a new assay coming into service or instrument replacements. To reiterate: the only time you can be absolutely confident of your results is after you participate and complete in an inter-laboratory comparison program.

If your laboratory has a history of no discrepancies on your inter-laboratory comparison program(s), you need to investigate why? *All* quality laboratories have discrepancies in inter-laboratory comparison results. When discrepancies are identified, this is a real opportunity for improvement.

The first thing you need to do when investigating PT discrepancies is to review for clerical errors. You should examine the Discrepancy Report and all documentation and worksheets (paper and electronic). Evaluate if all the units were reported correctly, if the decimal point was entered into the correct place, were there accurate records of which peer group should be used for comparison, and whether there was a transcription error. A great many PT discrepancies are actually reporting errors.

If the paperwork is problem free, the next thing to do is to check available data on or about the time the PT sample was tested. What was the calibration status? Were patient results trending high or low? How about QC trends or major instrument maintenance/repairs? Who was doing the testing that day? As you move forward in your investigation, every puzzle piece counts.

We always recommend you save excess PT materials. Preferably, store them in the freezer to keep them as stable as possible, and also so you can retest them to compare results with those already reported. This alone could solve the mystery. Remember, however, that many PT samples are shipped without preservatives because they are designed to mimic normal patient samples as closely as possible and avoid, for example, the matrix effect. For this and other reasons, all PT samples stored for long periods of time prior to re-testing should be considered suspect.

The laboratory's performance for any PT challenge that was intended to be graded but was not, for any reason, needs to be evaluated by the laboratory. No matter what the cause for the inability to be graded (e.g., lack of consensus, delay in returning the laboratory's analysis), the laboratory must determine if its performance is acceptable or not. If not acceptable, the laboratory must perform a root-cause analysis just as it would for a graded, missed challenge.

If your investigation finds a systemic problem, you may need to review your patient results to see if any were affected. This should be done in conjunction with the medical director. If reported results were invalid, you will need to recall those results.

After you investigate a discrepant PT result, you will need to report your findings and detail the problem, including all investigation steps taken. If you discovered nothing, you will need to report this as an outlier or random error and henceforth pay special attention to the future performance of this assay. Note that this conclusion can only be reached when you exclude all other potential causes.

Multiple sequential PT failures may be the result of a systemic failure in your laboratory, and the situation needs to be disclosed, discussed, and forward action determined at the highest level. This forward action may include ceasing testing and sending the assay to a referral laboratory until the problem is resolved.

Why being in compliance with this FOS is important:

Internal quality control is done within the isolation of your own laboratory systems. If there are fundamental problems in these internal systems, and you do not check this with external comparisons, it is possible you are reporting suboptimal results forever. We have, in fact, seen this occur where a laboratory reported out more than 200,000 results over a decade with a 20% negative bias. They (and especially the new quality manager) were pretty shocked when they did their first inter-laboratory comparison.

Materials Included In This FOS
• Inter-Laboratory Comparisons Policies and Procedures
• Inter-Laboratory Comparison Program Plan
• Inter-Laboratory Comparisons Evaluation

FOS: Nonconformities / ISO 4.9, 4.10, 4.11

4.9 Identification and Control of Nonconformities

The laboratory shall have a documented procedure to identify and manage nonconformities in any aspect of the quality management system, including pre-examination, examination, or post-examination processes.

The procedure shall ensure that:

a) The responsibilities and authorities for handling nonconformities are designated;
b) The immediate actions to be taken are defined;
c) The extent of the nonconformity is determined;
d) Examinations are halted and reports withheld as necessary;
e) The medical significance of any nonconforming examination is considered and, where applicable, the requesting clinician or authorized individual responsible for using the results is informed;
f) The results of any nonconformities or potentially nonconforming examinations already are recalled or appropriately identified, as necessary;
g) The responsibility for authorization of the resumption of examinations is defined;
h) Each episode of nonconformity is documented and recorded, with these records being reviewed at regular specified intervals to detect trends and initiate corrective action.

NOTE: Nonconforming examinations or activities occur in many different areas and can be identified in many different ways, including clinician complaints, internal quality control indications, instrument calibrations, checking for consumable materials, inter-laboratory comparison, staff comments, reporting and certificate checking, laboratory management reviews, and internal and external audits.

When it is determined that nonconformities in pre-examination, examination and post-examination processes could recur or that there is doubt about the laboratory's compliance with its own procedures, the laboratory shall take action to identify, document and eliminate the cause(s).

Corrective action to be taken shall be determined and documented (see 4.10).

4.10 Corrective Action

The laboratory shall take corrective action to eliminate the cause(s) of nonconformities.

Corrective actions shall be appropriate to the effects of the nonconformities encountered.

The laboratory shall have documented procedures for:

a) Reviewing nonconformities;
b) Determining the root cause of nonconformities;
c) Evaluating the need for corrective action to ensure that nonconformities do not recur;
d) Determining and implementing corrective action needed;
e) Recording the results of corrective action taken (see 4.14.5);
f) Reviewing the effectiveness of the corrective action taken (see 4.15).

NOTE: Action taken at the time of the nonconformity to mitigate its immediate effects is considered "immediate action". Only action taken to remove the root cause of the problem that is causing the nonconformities is considered "corrective action".

4.11 Preventative Action

The laboratory shall determine action to eliminate the causes of potential nonconformities in order to prevent their occurrence. Preventative actions shall be appropriate to the effects of the potential problems.

The laboratory shall have a documented procedure for:

a) Reviewing laboratory data and information to determine where potential nonconformities exist;
b) Determining the root cause(s) of potential nonconformities;
c) Evaluating the need for preventative action to prevent the occurrence of nonconformities;

d) Determining and implementing preventative action needed;
e) Recording the results of preventative action taken (see 4.13);
f) Reviewing the effectiveness of the preventative action taken.

NOTE: Preventative action is a proactive process for identifying opportunities for improvement rather than a reaction to the identification of a problem or complaints (i.e., nonconformities). In addition to review of the operation procedures, preventative action might involve analysis of data, including trend and risk analyses and external quality assessment (proficiency testing).

REMARKS

Basically, what is being asked of you here is:

a) To adhere to your own policies and procedures
b) To have ways of ensuring you are adhering to your own policies and procedures
c) When you discover you are not complying with your own policies and procedures, to have some documented way of returning to compliance
d) When you find you are not complying with your own policies and procedures, determine if damage had been done and perform corrective action, if necessary
e) Identify ways to proactively make sure you do not violate your own policies and procedures

You can identify nonconformities the hard or easy way. The hard way refers to situations where some kind of nonconformity causes harm, and you must deal with, not only correcting the nonconformity, but the consequences of the harm as well. The easy way would be identifying a nonconformity during an internal or external audit. There is also a best way—remaining in compliance with your policies and procedures at all times to minimize the occurrence of nonconformities.

The goal of staying in constant compliance is obvious; at the same time, it can be challenging. Luckily, you are a LEAP user. If you set up your QMS Maintenance properly and your Task Managers respond to email remainders and/or vigilantly monitor their personal My Tasks page, you can stay in compliance 24/7.

Why being in compliance with this FOS is important:

All too often, laboratory errors are not single failures to follow procedures. Rather, they tend to get baked into the system with inadequate procedures or systematic practices of not following them. For example, if your normal range is shifted and this shift was not recognized when it occurred, the results for all patients can get reported in error for extended periods of time. Even something as simple as a single non-calibrated pipette can reverberate throughout your laboratory in unpredictable ways. Identifying nonconformities quickly and dealing with them effectively is the hallmark of every quality laboratory. Your ability to do this well will impact your productivity, your staff, and the quality of patient care.

Materials Included In This FOS
• Nonconformities Policies and Procedures
• Nonconformity Event Reporting Form
• Nonconformity Event Investigation Log

FOS: Validation & Verification of Examination Procedures / ISO 5.5, 5.5.1, 5.5.1.1, 5.5.1.2, 5.5.1.3, 5.5.1.4, 5.5.2

5.5 Examination Processes

5.5.1 Selection, Verification and Validation of Examination Procedures

5.5.1.1 General

The laboratory shall select examination procedures, which have been validated for their intended use.

The identity of persons performing activities in examination processes shall be recorded.

The specific requirements (performance specifications) for each examination procedure shall relate to the intended use of that examination.

NOTE: Preferred procedures are those specified in the instructions for use of *in vitro* medical devices or those that have been published in established/ authoritative textbooks, peer-reviewed texts or journals, or in international consensus standards or guidelines, or in national or regional regulations.

5.5.1.2 Verification of Examination Procedures

Validated examination procedures used without modification shall be subject to independent verification by the laboratory before being introduced into routine use.

The laboratory shall obtain information from the manufacturer/method developer for confirming the performance characteristics of the procedure.

The independent verification by the laboratory shall confirm, through obtaining objective evidence (in the form of performance characteristics) that the performance claims for the examination procedure have been met. The performance claims for the examination procedure confirmed during the verification process shall be those relevant to the intended use of the examination results.

The laboratory shall document the procedure used for the verification and record results obtained. Staff with the appropriate authority shall review the verification results and record the review.

5.5.1.3 Validation of Examination Procedures

The laboratory shall validate examination procedures derived from the following sources:

a) Non-standard methods;
b) Laboratory designed or developed methods;
c) Standard methods used outside their intended scope;
d) Validated methods subsequently modified.

The validation shall be as extensive as is necessary and confirm, through the provision of objective evidence (in the form of performance characteristics), that the specific requirements for the intended use of the examination have been fulfilled.

NOTE: Performance characteristics of an examination procedure should include consideration of: measurement trueness; measurement accuracy; measurement precision including measurement repeatability and measurement intermediate precision; measurement uncertainty; analytical specificity including interfering substances, analytical sensitivity, detection limit and quantitation limit; measuring interval; diagnostic specificity; and diagnostic sensitivity.

The laboratory shall document the procedure used for the validation and record the results obtained. Staff with the appropriate authority shall review the validation and record the review.

When changes are made to a validated examination procedure, the influence of such changes shall be documented and, when appropriate, a new validation shall be carried out.

5.5.1.4 Measurement Uncertainty of Measured Quantity Values

The laboratory shall determine measurement uncertainty for each measurement procedure in the examination phase used to report measured quantity values on patients' samples.

The laboratory shall define the performance requirements for the measurement uncertainty of each measurement procedure and regularly review estimates of measurement uncertainty.

NOTE 1: The relevant uncertainties components are those associated with the actual measurement process, commencing with the presentation of the sample to the measurement procedure and ending with the output of the measure value.

NOTE 2: Measurement uncertainties may be calculated using quantity values obtained by the measurement of quality control materials under intermediate precision conditions that include as many routine changes as reasonably possible in the standard operation of a measurement procedure, e.g., changes of reagent and calibrator batches, different operators, scheduled instrument maintenance.

NOTE 3: Examples of the practical utility of measurement uncertainty estimates might include confirmation that patients' values meet quality goals set by the laboratory and meaningful comparison of a patient value with a previous value of the same type or with a clinical decision value.

The laboratory shall consider measurement uncertainty when interpreting measured quantity values.

Upon request, the laboratory shall make its estimates of measurement uncertainty available to laboratory users.

Where examinations include a measurement step but do not report a measured quantity value, the laboratory should calculate the uncertainty of the measurement step where its utility is assessing the reliability of the examination procedure or has influence on the reported result.

5.5.2 Biological Reference Intervals or Clinical Decision Values

The laboratory shall define the biological reference intervals or clinical decision values, document the basis for the reference intervals or decision values and communicate this information to the users.

When a particular biological reference interval or decision value is no longer relevant for the population served, appropriate changes shall be made and communicated to the users.

When the laboratory changes an examination procedure or pre-examination procedure, the laboratory shall review associated reference intervals and clinical decision values, as applicable.

REMARKS

The process of validation and verification is essential for ensuring examinations are performing to specification and providing users with information they need to accurately diagnose and treat patients. In general terms, there are two kinds of validation and verification processes: a) kits that have been pre-validated by an external manufacturer; and b) assays that are made in your laboratory (Laboratory Developed Tests: LDT). Kits that have been pre-validated by an external manufacturer for which you have deviated the process approved by that manufacturer must be treated as LDT.

If testing procedures are manufactured by another company and approved by a regulatory body (if required by local laws), the validation procedure (sometimes referred to as verification) needs to include the reagents as well as any other equipment or materials used in the examination process. While it is understood that manufacturers do their best to validate their products to their published specifications, they are ultimately not responsible for the welfare of patients. Therefore, in order to obtain and maintain accreditation, the laboratory itself is responsible for verifying that the assay systems are working to specification in your environment, with your equipment and with your personnel.

In case you are developing your own testing methodologies, the importance of validating and verifying those procedures prior to testing patients is even more important. If you choose to develop your own procedures (i.e., LDTs), for all intents and purposes, you will be required to take all steps required by a manufacturer of analytical systems. The methods vary depending upon technology and are beyond the scope of this book. However, most of the validation and verification procedures outlined here will apply.

The following is a list of validation and verification procedures which need to be taken for all assays prior to initiating patient testing:

a) Linearity and Analytical Measurement Range (AMR)/Dynamic Range
b) Precision (sometimes referred to as repeatability)
c) Accuracy
d) Correlation with Other Instruments or Methodologies
e) Interfering Substances Validation
f) Reportable Clinical Decision Values/Biological Reference Intervals
g) Measurement Uncertainty (MU)
h) Specimen Storage, Stability and Transportation Requirements
i) Dilution and Concentration Procedures (if applicable)

Simple examples of procedures have been included in this FOS, but please note that these procedures will vary depending upon the science and method of each examination and can be especially challenging in case of LDTs. Ensure that your thresholds for acceptability are established and documented before evaluating validation results, which should also be recorded. You are encouraged to consult CLSI guidelines.

Measurement Uncertainty (MU) is a relatively new concept for clinical laboratories and may be difficult to understand. You are encouraged to go to the following article for a complete and easy-to-understand explanation:

https://www.westgard.com/hitchhike-mu.htm

The laboratory director is ultimately responsible for approving these validations and authorizing their release for patient testing.

Why being in compliance with this FOS is important:

Validating and verifying your procedures both initially and after potentially impactful events can better assure the laboratory is not reporting aberrant results. It is noteworthy that these biases and aberrant results tend to be inherent in laboratory processes and may persist for long periods of time, impacting scores of patients, the reputation of the laboratory, and possible legal challenges.

Properly validating and verifying your procedures allows you to report results with confidence, knowing that you have confirmed, by all reasonable means, that the results reported are within your established tolerance limits. Remember, the laboratory is responsible for the quality of results, not the manufacturer of the instruments or reagent systems.

Materials Included In This FOS
• Validation and Verification of Examination Procedures Policies and Procedures
• Personnel Authorized to Confirm Validation and Verification Results
• Linearity and Analytical Measurement Range (AMR)/Dynamic Range Studies
• Linearity Calculation Worksheet
• Precision Studies
• Precision Calculation Worksheet
• Correlation Studies
• Interfering Substances Validation Studies
• Reportable Clinical Decision Values/Biological Reference Intervals Validation Studies
• Measurement Uncertainty (MU)

AUDIT

FOS: Audit Preparation

If your laboratory has gone through the process of building LEAP one FOS at a time, and you have reviewed all the information in the **FOS Content Library** and ensured that your laboratory staff members have reviewed and understood all the policies and procedures set up for each FOS as well as the LEAP Education Tools—you are ready for an audit.

To prepare for an audit, make sure both the LEAP **QMS Dashboard** and **Maintenance Dashboard** are green/yellow (i.e., ready-for-inspection) and refer to the Audit Preparation Checklist to ensure all tasks related to audit preparation are completed.

If you choose to, and if your assigned auditor is amenable, you can provide him/her with a LEAP account and password. This will allow them to review all materials saved on LEAP prior to and while inspecting your site, allowing for a more time efficient audit inspection.

Once your audit is complete, you can use LEAP to perform any corrections using one of the following methods:

1) For minor changes (e.g., missing signatures, missing dates), you can edit the MEF to modify materials accordingly. Once uploaded, the MEF should be re-submitted for approval to assure ongoing compliance by using LEAP maintenance protocols.
   For major changes, you must educate your staff members on the revised modifications; in such cases, the above method should **NOT** be an option.

If there are major changes, the following methods should be used:

2) If only one or a few FOSs in a certain department requires modification, a Gap Analysis can be done for non-compliant FOSs. You should answer "No" for FOSs with deficiencies pointed out during the audit, which will trigger LEAP to archive all documents currently saved for that

particular FOS and force you to rebuild the FOS according to the desired specifications.

3) If a department has more than a few deficiencies and an extensive change is required, a Self-Audit can be triggered for that particular department. Doing so will force department staff members to review all completed projects in the department and make the necessary modifications according to the desired specifications.

Know that, in many ways, ISO 15189 and CAP are a "guideline" on how to best approach QMS. LEAP was created to reduce deficiencies by taking a holistic approach. In the event that deficiencies are sited, simply correct these according to the direction of the ISO auditor and make sure these corrective actions are recorded.

Lastly, if you disagree with an auditor, it is within the rules to challenge their findings. If you find yourself in this position, address the issues respectfully and professionally and accept the final judgment of the accreditation body.

AUTHORS AND CONTRIBUTORS

Authors (Alphabetical Order)

Masahiko Amano, Ph.D.
Dr. Amano received his Ph.D. from the University of Alabama in Bio-Medical Engineering and did his post-doctoral work at Stanford University. He served as a research scientist at Mead-Toppan and was the technical supervisor for Next-Generation Sequence testing for Riken Genisis. Dr. Amano is the head engineer for the development of LEAP system content architecture and is involved in the implementation and maintenance of QMS in several large clinical and research laboratories.

Robert Bredt, M.D.
Dr. Robert Bredt, MD, is a board-certified pathologist/cytopathologist with extensive experience in quality and regulation. He has directed eight laboratories over his 25-year career in pathology and is currently medical director for the Texas Medical Board. He has lead and performed hundreds of inspections with CAP, served on the CAP Inspection Processes Committee, and now serves as the Southwest regional commissioner with CAP. Additionally, Dr. Bredt has performed many ISO 15189 accreditation assessments with the American Association of Laboratory Accreditation (A2LA), sits on the A2LA MedTAC Committee, and on the A2LA Accreditation Council. Dr. Bredt also serves as a consultant and lecturer on ISO 15159 and CLIA surveys.

Mark Colby, B.S.
Mark Colby is credited with introducing quality systems to clinical laboratories in Japan. He was the first to introduce both the College of American Pathologists (CAP) and the ISO 15189 standards. He is the founder and CEO of CGI KK, a company that specializes in helping clinical laboratories gain and maintain QMS through the implementation of advanced software systems. Colby is the author of numerous books and papers on healthcare policy and business and is the editor-and-chief of the periodical, *Invitro Diagnostic Global News.*

Trent Freeman, B.S. M.A, MT (ASCP)CT
Mr. Freeman received his MA from Webster University and BS from Excelsior College and was Assistant Professor of Clinical Research and Leadership, Medical Laboratory Science, George Washington University. He is a retired US Naval Officer with the rank of Lt. Commander. In the Navy he was the Division Officer, Core Laboratory & Complex Testing, Naval Medical Center San Diego, Division Officer, Blood Bank & Quality and Department Head, Naval Hospital Yokosuka, Japan. Mr. Freeman now serves as Senior Manager, University of Texas Health System, and is a black belt in Lean Six Sigma as well as an experienced QMS inspector of clinical laboratories.

Contributors (Alphabetical Order)

Minami Alevoet-Eto, B.S.
Minami Alevoet-Eto is a graduate of University of Virginia with a bachelor's degree in Molecular Biology. Ms. Alevoet-Eto has worked as a technical translator and interpreter for clinical laboratory specialties and has supported the College of American Pathologists' inspection process. She was the lead contributor in the development of the final work-product content for the LEAP software as it pertains to ISO 15189 as well as much of the final processes described in this book.

Sean Crownover, B.S.
Sean Crownover has a bachelor's degree in computer science from San Francisco State University. He has worked for over 20 years developing advanced software solutions, including cloud computing and Software-as-a-Service (SaaS) systems. Sean coordinated the development of this book's content, ensuring it is congruent with the parameters set forth in the LEAP systems.

Masataka Kawagoe, B.S., M.S.
Mr. Kawagoe is a graduate of Kyushu University with a master's degree in bio-engineering. He worked in the Teijin group and founded and ran the joint venture clinical laboratory between Teijin and Dow Chemical called Teijin Bio Laboratories, where he served as laboratory director, leading the laboratory through the College of American Pathologists (CAP) accreditation programs. Mr. Kawagoe is also in expert in ISO systems, managing the implementation of ISO programs throughout the Teijin group worldwide. He is currently the business unit manager for CGI's CAP accreditation and ISO 15189 SaaS support programs.

Marcus Houston, M.T.
Marcus Houston has operated and managed clinical laboratories for over 20 years while serving in the United States Air Force. His areas of specialities are the blood bank, clinical chemistry, and microbiology testing. Mr. Houston is an expert in the validation and quality control processes for all areas of clinical testing. He was a valuable contributor for all aspects of developing and fact-checking the contents of this book.

Tsukasa Narita, B.S., M.T.
Mr. Narita is a graduate of Kitazato University and is a licensed medical technologist. He served as the chief medical technologist at Aizu General Hospital and later became the head medical technologist at Hoken Kagaku East Clinical Reference Laboratory where he also sat on the board of directors. Mr. Narita lead his laboratory through both the College of American Pathologists (CAP) and ISO 15189 accreditation process. He is a qualified ISO 15189 inspector and currently specializes in teaching laboratories how to best implement ISO 15189 processes.

Masahisa Takeda, M.S.
Mr. Takeda received his master's degree in molecular biology from Jichi University. He served as the head of the molecular pathology department at LSI Medi-science Clinical Laboratory and is now the head of CGI's group aiding molecular pathology and specialty laboratories through the College of American Pathologists, CLIA, and ISO 15189 processes. Mr. Takeda has been instrumental in the development of technical content for LEAP software systems.

Hiromitsu Tazawa, M.S.
Mr. Tazawa received his masters of science degree from Okayama University and was the chief medical technologist at Sumitomo Medals BioScience and later served on the board of directors. He also oversaw the implementation of The College of American Pathologists (CAP) and ISO 15189 Quality Management Systems. Other posts include the CEO of SRL Laboratories and was the Executive Officer of Miraca Holdings. He is currently the President of KBBM Inc., a newly founded bio-venture company.

Steve Ziolkowski, M.A.
Born in Montreal, Quebec, Steve Ziolkowski was educated in Canada, the U.K. and US. Steve has taught at a broad range of institutions in Canada, Japan, and Taiwan and has lived in five countries. He was Managing Director of Oxford University Press, Japan and has authored or edited over 20 books. For the last two decades, Steve has managed his own communications company, TransPac. He also sits on the board of a US software company and a Japanese PR firm.

Acknowledgments

Cover Illustration: Mark A. Colby
Project Management: TransPac Communications
Book Layout and Design: Greg Glover
Publishing Consulting: Mark Gresham, MHM
Index: Word Tapestries, Inc.
Editorial Liaison: Joy Quek, World Scientific

INDEX

H

I

J

L

M

N

O

P

Q

R

S

T